ABIGAIL S. HARDIN, PH.D.

The COVID-19 Survival Guide

*How to Prepare for, Manage, and Overcome a
Coronavirus Infection*

First edition

This book was professionally typeset on Reedsy.
Find out more at reedsy.com

This book is dedicated to the survivors of COVID-19, whose words of wisdom and stories you will find quoted throughout this book. This book is also dedicated to those on their journey of rehabilitation from any serious illness or injury. Finally, this book is for all those with disabilities of any kind. May we one day create a society of love, respect and inclusion.

Contents

Acknowledgement

Thank you to Seth Zehler who graciously and lovingly cooked, cleaned and maintained our entire household when I launched this project and fell off the face of the earth. Not only did he keep me fed throughout this endeavor, but he patiently listened to my ideas and provided helpful feedback without once muttering under his breath about the ever-growing laundry pile. He cheered me on tirelessly, and I deeply appreciate it. I promise I will start doing the laundry again, Seth.

Thank you also to Dr. Alisha Janssen, who contributed ideas, comments and feedback from her personal work in rehabilitation and with COVID-19 survivors and healthcare staff. True friendship is being able to say "your sentence construction here is awful" and still love each other afterward. Dr. Janssen is now, and always will be, both a professional and personal role model to me who shows warmth and charm to all those she encounters. Thanks for being my friend, Dr. Janssen.

Finally, I'd like to thank my mother, Deanna Strom, who has been my tireless writing coach and line editor since about age 9, and without whom I would still not understand transitive verbs. Ok fine, I still don't understand transitive verbs. Thanks for putting up with me, Mom.

Introduction

"I wish people would realize how many of us have lasting significant problems as a result of this virus—even healthy people! I run 100-mile races, but COVID-19 brought me to my knees. Once you get exposed, it may affect your health for a very long time. And the symptoms come in waves. I was very careful and I still got COVID-19."
- Karen

The pandemic brought on by the coronavirus has swept the globe and impacted every one of us. It has changed how we travel, shop at the market, and go to the dentist. It has shaped how we work and interact with loved ones. It has made many of us worried—about infection, our health, and the lives already lost. And this fear is very understandable—there are still many unknowns about COVID-19, despite the tireless efforts of scientists and doctors to conduct research and create a vaccine. What we do know is that COVID-19 can cause serious illness leading to hospitalization, intensive care unit admission, and death in people of any age.

Your worries might be: *What do I do if I test positive? What will happen to me? Will I have to go to the hospital? What will treatments look like? What are my chances of survival? Will I have a long recovery? Will I be the same again? How do I deal with long-term effects? How do I support someone who has the virus?*

If any of these questions have ever crossed your mind, this book is for you. I have worked with hundreds of patients—and their loved ones—who've expressed these same questions, and I've helped walk many through the entire COVID-19 experience. Now I can help you, too.

I am a licensed clinical psychologist who specializes in a type of practice called rehabilitation psychology. I specialize in working with people who have sustained catastrophic illnesses and injuries, with a particular emphasis on those who have survived intensive care unit admissions. I have been providing direct care to COVID-19 patients since the beginning of the pandemic, including follow-up care months after their discharge from the hospital. I have worked in some of the best hospitals and rehabilitation centers in the U.S., and my job is to help people in the hospital make the most of their recoveries, no matter how catastrophic their illness or injury has been. I work with patients to ensure that after they have survived, they can thrive.

This book was born one evening when I came home from a long day of working with COVID-19 survivors on my rehabilitation unit. A growing sense of disquiet had been building in me for some time, and as I sat on my couch trying to decompress, it finally detonated into full-blown fear. It was clear to me, even in the early days of the pandemic, that many survivors of COVID-19 would experience long-term symptoms. Between the intensity of the COVID-19 surge and the fact that people like me who specialize in recovery from critical illness are few and far between, I realized hundreds of thousands of COVID-19 survivors across the U.S. would be leaving hospitals and clinics without the education, rehabilitation and treatment they would need. That thought terrified me. Though the U.S. healthcare system is pretty good at saving lives, it is pretty terrible, even in the best of times, at adequately addressing emotional concerns, and it was proving particularly unprepared at dealing with the additional cognitive and physical impacts of long-haul COVID-19 symptoms. I realized that while I would like to be in every hospital at once providing this guidance to all who need it, I simply couldn't. So, I wrote this book to act as an extension of myself so that everyone, everywhere can receive the practical guidance they need to survive COVID-19 and thrive after, even in the presence of long-haul symptoms.

How This Book Can Help

You don't have to face COVID-19, hospitals, doctors, acute rehabilitation, or adjusting back to "normal" on your own. Whether you are healthy and just want to be prepared for the disease, are currently sick with COVID-19, are already in recovery, or are caring for someone with the virus, this book is for you.

The truth is, most people, not even healthcare workers, fully understand how the healthcare system works. Even the brightest among us can struggle with how best to navigate the process of being hospitalized, recovering, and getting home. It frustrates me, as a healthcare provider, to see families getting lost in the healthcare system, slipping between the cracks and going home without all the information or care they need.

This book will offer support and guidance as you go through the process so you can manage the infection and return to wellness, work, and your loved ones sooner.

I hope you never get COVID-19. But if you or someone in your family does, this book will teach you:

- How to protect yourself from and prepare for COVID-19
- What symptoms you might get and how to best manage them
- What to do if it's time to go to the hospital
- How to navigate the hospitalization process
- How to work with the medical team to get the best care possible
- What to expect during COVID-19 rehabilitation and how to set and reach goals
- What you can do to make the most of your survival and recovery so you can return to a life that is meaningful

> *"I want to shout at people from the rooftops, 'This is not a hoax! This is not the flu!' This is not something that will just go away. This is not something that only affects the elderly or the immunocompromised. This virus affects everyone. Show Compassion. Show Love. Show how much we care about each other and this nation.'"*
> - Danielle

Survival is just the beginning

If you need to be hospitalized, a team of healthcare professionals will be administering treatments and medications intended to save your life. They will help monitor your blood pressure, blood oxygen content (oxygenation), and a whole host of other things in order to treat you and keep you alive. That's your number-one goal: to survive. Even if you never go to the hospital, your objective is the same.

Whether you receive intensive care or not, I want you to not only survive your diagnosis, I want you to thrive afterward. That may seem simplistic, but for some patients and their loved ones, getting back on their feet and enjoying life again is a long and difficult process. On top of learning to walk or breathe again, you may also struggle with depression or trauma symptoms—even months after a negative test. Remember, survival is not the end. Survival is just the beginning.

Every day I help families answer questions about COVID-19:

- What can I do before I get sick to prepare?
- How can my family help me while I'm in the hospital?
- How will my family and I manage the tremendous stress that comes along with being critically ill?
- How will I keep track of the necessary paperwork?
- How can I ensure I'm getting the best rehabilitation and make sure my recovery goes as well as possible?
- How do I know which healthcare professionals to see?
- How can I cope afterward with any long-term symptoms?
- How can I successfully transition back into a meaningful life after surviving COVID-19?

"The panic of contracting a virus that is basically untreatable and is so new is unbelievably stressful."
- Misty

The answers to all of these questions and more are found in

that's how scientists arrived at that name.

Generally, this type of virus causes mild symptoms in humans,[2] but there have been two coronaviruses like COVID-19 that have caused more severe illness in humans. Those include SARS, in 2002 and Middle East Respiratory Syndrome (MERS) in 2012.[2]

COVID-19 appears to be passed through small droplets in the air that are expelled when someone who is infected coughs, or sneezes.[3] Anyone of any age can get sick, and those who don't even have symptoms can spread the disease.[4] These droplets that contain the virus are the reason why wearing masks and staying six feet apart or more is recommended to prevent transmission of the disease.

What are the symptoms?

COVID-19, according to the information currently available, kills about 2% of people who get it.[5] The early symptoms of COVID-19 include fever, dry cough and shortness of breath.[6] New evidence also seems to show loss of smell/taste might be a symptom.[7]

> *"My early symptoms were feeling a bit disoriented, loss of smell, sore throat and chest pain like [I] was being poked hard. The scariest part was struggling to get enough air to dry cough, this lasted about 24hrs with a very high temperature".*
> - Deb

> *"I had a runny nose and cough for most of the winter. I was training for a 100m race and doing well so it wasn't*

debilitating. On March 21 my long run felt hard and so I stopped at mile 13ish. The next day when I made my morning coffee I thought the machine made a bad cup because it tasted like hot brown water. Weird, I thought to myself. Later that afternoon I made a pot of soup. While chopping the onion I noticed that it had no aroma. What a strange onion, I thought to myself. Later that night I was scrolling through news stories and came across an article from England that was reporting on loss of smell as a symptom of COVID-19! (This was not yet common knowledge here in the states.) When I read that article, I jumped up and tried smelling soaps that I knew had scents. Nothing!! I knew I had COVID-19".

- Karen

The symptoms don't stop after survival. Even months after patients leave the hospital, symptoms are still problematic.[8] In one recent research study of patients who had been critically ill with COVID-19 and housed in an intensive care unit (ICU), 72% experienced long-term fatigue, and 47% experienced long-term psychological distress. Even those who had less severe cases of COVID-19 and were never in the ICU experienced long-term symptoms. Of those who were in the hospital without ICU care, 60% experienced long-term fatigue and 42% experienced psychological distress.[8]

These findings have been replicated across the globe. In Italy, researchers followed patients after they left the hospital and found that even after seven weeks, more than half still complained of fatigue, 43% still had breathing issues, and 27% had joint pain.[9]

Another study showed that more than half of all COVID-

19 survivors studied had significant mental health concerns. These included depression, anxiety, obsessive-compulsive symptoms, PTSD and insomnia. Anxiety and insomnia were the most common symptoms in survivors.[10]

> *"I had to be separated from my husband and isolated and after 6 days my oxygen level rose enough to finally bring me out of a critical status. It was one of the most terrifying experiences, physically and emotionally because I knew how close I was to dying and I heard the codes all around me in the hospital of people who didn't make it. My husband thankfully recovered quickly. Here I am now, five months later with residual issues including the extra heart beats, tachycardia [rapid heart rate], telogen effluvium [hair loss] and fatigue to name a few. I want people to understand this is real and how dehumanizing it is to see that there are still so many who think it is a hoax or a flu."*
> - Wendy

Researchers are still looking into how people recover from COVID-19, but the data we have so far suggest that even well after you survive COVID-19, physical and psychological problems continue. This means that survival is only the first part of the battle.

> *"I hope people would know that this affects people in many different ways and with varying severity/intensity. Symptoms may linger for months."*
> - Isaiah

What is not clear right now is why these symptoms linger. You'll see in Chapter 5, "If you become critically ill" that illnesses, even those other than COVID-19, can cause a set of common but profound problems that last months after discharge from the hospital. Many people in the media have said that the long-term effects seen in people who survive COVID-19 are "unprecedented", using hashtags like #longcovid and seeming to suggest that the lingering symptoms after recovery are entirely unexpected.

The fact is, the medical research literature has clearly documented for many years that there are common symptoms that persist after many critical illnesses, and not just COVID-19. Why so many medical professionals don't recognize these symptoms is a topic for another book entirely. But for you, the reader, it's important. This means that you'll need to be an advocate for yourself in a U.S. healthcare system that is likely to overlook your long-term symptoms, while also navigating the unique experience of having a novel disease that many physicians do not understand well. It's a recipe for anxiety and uncertainty.

At the same time, because COVID-19 is so new, it's not yet understood what symptoms linger and why, and what may be going on "under the hood", so to speak, that causes long-term symptoms. It may be the case that some or even many of the long-term symptoms of COVID-19 turn out to be unique to this disease, while others may be very similar to those long-term symptoms we already understand. We just don't know yet. But there is already enough information from similar diseases and the symptoms they cause for you to use the information in this book to help you navigate your recovery process effectively. So, use this book to arm yourself with knowledge that will help you advocate for yourself and your family members so you don't slip through the cracks of our broken healthcare system.

Are you at risk?

"I awoke on March 30 and noticed immediately that I couldn't catch my breath. My nose felt congested and swollen and my breathing was coming in short and fast, gasping breaths like someone had put a plastic bag over my head, tightened it, pinched the top of my nose and poked a needle through the plastic bag near my mouth so I could get the shortest breath in and out; fast and shallow breaths. I stood up to go to the washroom and I almost fell to the floor...I had heard about COVID-19. I wasn't too concerned...I am a 39-year-old healthy woman."
- Jeness

It's odd – it seems COVID-19 affects some patients very severely, and others may never know they had it. What sets these groups apart? In one early study of Chinese patients, 91% of hospitalized COVID-19 patients (meaning, they had a fairly serious case), had some type of additional underlying health problem.[11] High blood pressure was the most common underlying health problem, but other problems included diabetes and heart disease. People who were older were more likely to die in the hospital of COVID-19.[11]

Additionally, in another study, obesity was a risk factor for having a more severe COVID-19 case, even after researchers accounted for underlying health conditions like high blood pressure, high blood lipids, diabetes, age, sex, and smoking.[12]

A later, larger study found roughly the same thing again:

older age, heart disease, diabetes, obesity, chronic lung disease, high blood pressure and cancer were all connected to a greater chance of death from COVID-19.[13]

But these are just group statistics. Plenty of people without an underlying health condition can, and have, died or had severe consequences from COVID-19. What's more, nearly half of adults in the U.S. have high blood pressure.[14] Combine this with the fact that 42.5% of people in the U.S. meet criteria for obesity (defined as a body mass index greater than 25), there is a very good chance you, or someone you know, is at risk.[15]

Now that you understand this disease and the risks to you and your family, it's time to prepare. Many people find thinking about their own vulnerability to disease, whether it is COVID-19 or something else, completely overwhelming. As a result, they stick their heads in the metaphorical sand, and fail to take even simple steps that would keep themselves safe or prepare themselves in a worst case scenario. I understand this urge to avoid discomfort and fear; sometimes I avoid things I'm scared of too. But in any challenge, there are those who collapse in fear, there are those who pretend not to be afraid and act rashly, and then there are those who study and prepare. Who do you think has the best results? Who do you want to be?

2

Preparing your family

Staying safe and avoiding COVID-19

Prevention strategies backed by science

According to the Centers for Disease Control, these are the only scientifically-supported methods for keeping yourself safe from COVID-19:[16]

- *Wash your hands.* Wash your hands often, especially after eating, touching food, leaving a public place, blowing your nose/coughing, changing a diaper, touching someone else, touching an animal, before touching your face, or after using the restroom. Use soap and water to wash your hands for at least 20 seconds (or about how long it takes to sing the "Happy Birthday" song twice).
- *Sanitize if needed.* If soap and water aren't available, use an alcohol-based hand sanitizer (60% alcohol or more).
- *Socially distance yourself.* Avoid close contact with people

– try to stay at least six feet apart, or more.
- **Wear a mask.** Wear a mask anytime you leave your house (except for very young children).
- **Keep things clean.** Clean and disinfect surfaces you touch frequently like countertops, handles, your phone, light switches, etc.

"This is what I tell everyone. Please be safe out there. Let's all do our part and wear a mask no matter where or who [we're] around. I don't want any of you to go through what I did...I want to be a cautionary tale for anyone not taking this virus seriously."
– Misty

That's it. That's the whole list. It seems like a pretty short list of actions you can take to help prevent such a serious disease. Many people anxiously feel as though they need to do more to protect themselves, and find themselves buying products advertised online, or following advice they read on Instagram. Remember, it is normal to feel anxiety and nervousness about something you can't control, like a global pandemic. And it is also normal to respond to that anxiety by wanting to take action to protect yourself and make yourself feel safer. But, doing the above behaviors are your absolute best shot at staying safe. Anything else you do is at best only impacting your risk a little, and at worst could be harmful, depending on what it is.

I will go over the purpose of each of these items in Chapter 4. For now, get your kit together so that you have it when you need it.

Getting paperwork in order

If you have been to the hospital before, you already know that paperwork is a big part of the hospitalization process. In the following chapters, you will find a few recommended documents that if possible, you should have for each adult in your family. If you don't already have these and you are healthy, take some time this weekend to start pulling these together. If you are already sick, there will be a social worker and/or case manager at the hospital who can help you.

Document 1: Advanced Directive

An advanced directive is a document that ensures your wishes are respected if for some reason you cannot make your own choices or direct your own care. When you are very sick, this can include situations like being sedated, intubated (put on a breathing machine), or otherwise mentally incapacitated. The advanced directive document, sometimes known as a "living will" outlines what kind of life saving care you want, or don't want. This is a legal document, and in order to be valid, it must be signed and witnessed. Depending on what U.S. state you live in, the form you use might be different. A simple way to get an advanced directive is to visit https://www.aarp.org/caregiving/financial-legal/free-printable-advance-directives and click on the name of your state. The document will provide you with exact instructions to complete your advanced directive and ensure it can be legally used if you get sick.

Another way to get an advanced directive is to work directly with your family's attorney, if you have one. If you are healthy as you read this, make sure you prioritize creating advanced directives for all the adults in your family.

If you do not create an advanced directive and you end up in the hospital unable to make your own decisions, you should know that the hospital will make the assumption that you want all available measures deployed to save your life. The hospital term for this is known as a "full code". Being labeled as "full code" includes measures like, but not limited to, bone-cracking chest compressions, defibrillation (shocking your heart), being mechanically ventilated on a breathing machine, having feeding tubes inserted, diversion of your intestines (known as a colostomy), and so on. Even just reading this list of life-saving measures can make most people see why it can be hard to create an advanced directive document. These are hard choices to make, and most of us would rather just not think about them.

But these conversations and choices are exactly why the hard part about making advanced directives is not actually the paperwork part (thank goodness). The hard part is sitting down with your loved ones and having this very difficult conversation about what you will want if you are very ill or dying. I know those are not fun discussions to have, and it's a lot easier to carry on assuming nothing bad will ever happen to us. But, I have two short stories (based on real-life couples I worked with) that may help you see why it's in your best interest, and in the best interest of those who love you, to have the hard conversation and complete your advanced directive.

First, take Mary and Bill, who have been married for 32 years. Bill felt uncomfortable at first talking to Mary about what care he wanted for himself if he were to get sick, so he just kept putting it off. As a cancer survivor, he knew he wanted to have some life-sustaining care, but he also knew he would never want to have extreme measures taken at his end-of-life, like having chest compressions that could crack his ribs, or a breathing tube. When Bill got sick, he wasn't able to make his own medical decisions, so his physicians called Mary to ask her what Bill would want, if his care should come to that. Mary didn't know, and she felt incredibly fearful that she would make the wrong choice. She called all of Bill's siblings, but they all seemed to have different ideas about what he would want. Fortunately, Bill survived his illness without Mary needing to make any decisions without Bill's input. Nonetheless, the experience was stressful and traumatic for Mary, the exact feelings that Bill was trying to prevent by delaying the discussion of his advanced directive!

Caitlin and Jeff's story has a similar theme. The two were newlyweds and in their prime of life. Jeff, however, was in a major car accident when he was 15, and since then has understood how important it is to have an advanced directive in place, in case of hospitalization. Jeff and Caitlin sat down one Sunday and created their legal advanced directives. They gave copies to their family members and their attorney. When Caitlin got injured, Jeff had the advanced directive ready, and gave it to his case manager at the hospital. Sadly, Caitlin died, but Jeff felt certain that her care was exactly as she wished. She died peacefully. While Jeff was grieving, one thing for which he felt very grateful was knowing he gave Caitlin the end of life experience she would have wanted. That made him feel like he had been a good husband to her.

Remember, advanced directives are hard to talk about for a few moments, but are a gift you give your loved ones to ensure they have peace of mind and clarity when they are helping you through your hospitalization. And should the worst happen, they leave your family members with the certainty that they did the right thing.

Document 2: Power of Attorney

A power of attorney (POA) is a document that lets you pick, in advance, who you want to act as your "agent" (the person who makes your decisions for you) in case you are incapacitated. There are multiple types of POAs, but for our purposes we will specifically focus on the healthcare POA. If you can't make your own decisions, or if you can't communicate them to your team (you're unconscious, for instance), the POA names someone you trust to make those decisions on your behalf. If you don't have a POA, your POA will automatically be someone closely related to you, depending on your state's laws. If you have an advanced directive, it should name your POA for healthcare matters. However, if you also want to name an agent to work on your behalf for say, financial matters (opening and closing accounts, authorizing real estate transactions, etc.) you may need a different type of POA.

It is important for you to know that if you don't establish a healthcare POA for yourself in advance, your medical decision making will be automatically assigned, based on your state of residence, to a family member or family members. If the decision legally falls to your siblings, they would all need to share and agree on decision-making equally. I have personally seen some very sticky situations in which family members had to equally share the immense responsibility of medical decision making and had trouble coming to a consensus, causing conflict and distress. This is why I advocate so strongly for setting a healthcare POA in advance.

An easy way to ensure you have your POAs completed is to go to https://powerofattorney.com and fill out the forms for the type of POA you want to have. There are multiple types, including durable POAs, financial POAs, etc. For the purposes of this book and for COVID-19, you'll want to ensure you have, at a minimum, an advanced directive and a healthcare POA.

Again, if you're healthy and have a family attorney, reach out to that person as soon as possible to start the process of getting these documents together.

Document 3: Will

A will is a document that details how you wish your property to be distributed after you die, and how to arrange care of your children if you die and they are still minors. Just like talking about advanced directives, talking about wills can be touchy, emotionally taxing, and stressful. But I promise, from seeing dozens of families struggle after the death of a loved one, it is so much better to get this done now than to force your family to struggle with it after you're gone.

"I couldn't breathe in fully no matter how hard I tried. I contacted my lawyer and put together a will as I realized how unprepared I was if I were to pass away."
- Jeness

LegalZoom and Quicken both make products you can buy to create your own will yourself. I have not used their products, and therefore cannot endorse them. They are options if you would rather not use an attorney. Another option would be to call your family attorney, if you have one. Additionally, many employers have a benefit available to employees that provides them with free legal advice up to a certain amount of time (usually 30 minutes or an hour per year). If you have this benefit, be sure to take advantage of it to create your will now, when you're healthy.

Other healthcare documents

In addition to the healthcare insurance and prescription coverage cards that you have in your COVID-19 kit, you will also want to gather up copies of your coverage information. Find out what type of coverage you have for emergency visits, hospital admissions, and rehabilitation. You will also want to know what type of coverage is available to you for aftercare. Find out how many days of acute rehabilitation (this is rehabilitation you do while still living in the hospital) your insurance will cover. Also ask if you have benefits for skilled nursing facilities, at-home nursing or rehabilitation (called "home health" services), and outpatient physical, occupational and speech therapies. Some individuals may also have a type of insurance called a "long-term care policy" that covers expenses associated with home caregivers, assisted living facilities and skilled nursing above and beyond what's covered by your basic medical insurance policy. If you have a policy like this, include it in your COVID-19 kit. While you're at it, find out what type of mental health care coverage you have for outpatient therapy.

If you are over 65 and have Medicare, you should also find out if you have Medicare Part A (hospital coverage), Part B (outpatient coverage), Part C (Medicare Advantage), Part D (prescription coverage) and whether you have some or all of these.

Once you have your advanced directive, POA, will, and health-care documents together, keep copies of all of these together in a single folder that you can easily find in case of a hospital admission. Lastly, make sure to inform your POA and family members where to find that folder in case you don't have time to grab it yourself.

Assessing your overall health

If you are reading this and you're healthy, there are things you can do now that might help if you end up getting COVID-19. Some of the troubling, long-term effects of COVID-19 are more likely to happen if you have a history of high blood pressure.[18] If you have high blood pressure or have been avoiding seeing your physician, this would be a good time to minimize your risk factors by monitoring your blood pressure and keeping up with your medications. Additionally, you may consider making one or several of the following health behavior changes:

- Quit smoking
- Eat nutritious, balanced meals
- Drink only moderately
- Get plenty of rest
- Manage chronic stress
- Get safe, socially distanced exercise

I will go over each of these health behavior changes below. As you read them, make note of what areas of your health you may want to change, and what areas you have already optimized.

Quit smoking

If you're a smoker, this is a fabulous time to quit. Smoking can increase your risk of viral infections like the common cold, and make your infection and ensuing illness more severe.[19] And, even though the science is still new, early results seem to suggest there is a link between smoking and COVID-19 severity.[20] I had one patient who told me the COVID-19 pandemic was the final push she needed to stop smoking permanently. Once she did, her smoker's cough vanished and now she feels safer knowing she has eliminated one of her risk factors, in case she gets COVID-19.

If you need help quitting smoking, google the name of your state and "quit smoking helpline" to get in touch with a free telephone helpline that can help you find resources to quit smoking. You can also make an appointment to see your primary care physician to request information on quitting aides, like nicotine patches and medications that might help. Many primary care clinics also offer co-located mental health professionals you can see for a short time to address things like quitting smoking.

Eat nutritious, balanced meals

The typical diet of the average U.S. citizen is referred to by scientists as the "Western Diet" and is characterized by excessive consumption of saturated fats, salt, added sugars, and an insufficient consumption of omega-3 fatty acids. There is substantial and damning evidence that the Western Diet harms immune function in humans.[21] So what diet is best? There is a myriad of very good online resources about healthy meal-planning. If you're new to healthy eating, there are two resources that make good starting points. The first is www.choosemyplate.gov, which has a two-week healthy eating menu along with basic information about healthy eating and micronutrients. The other is www.heart.org, which has good information on the Mediterranean Diet. The Mediterranean Diet has many health benefits, only one of which is that it supports a healthy immune system[22] thereby reducing the likelihood of viral infections.[23] Start with one or both of these two resources if you're new to healthy eating. Stay away from fad diets that involve fasting, only eating a certain type of food, cutting out entire food groups, or other extreme diets as these can substantially disrupt your immune system.

Drink only moderately

Drinking alcohol excessively can put you at greater risk of viral and bacterial infections of all kind, and if you are infected, make the severity of your infection worse.[24] This is true for COVID-19 too.[25] So, during the pandemic, it is recommended that you drink alcohol only in moderation. But how much is "moderate" alcohol use? For women, that means no more than one drink per day, and for men, no more than two drinks per day.[26]

If you are consuming alcohol heavily or are using hard drugs, you may consider cutting back, or quitting entirely. Reach out to your primary care physician and ask for a referral to your healthcare system's psychology department and/or substance abuse department if you need help quitting or have withdrawal symptoms when you try to quit.

Get plenty of rest

Not getting enough sleep can make you more susceptible to infections.[27] Also, once a vaccine is (hopefully) developed for COVID-19, getting good rest around the time you're vaccinated is a smart choice, as sleep is associated with improved immune reactions to vaccinations.[28] If you're drinking alcohol to help yourself drift to sleep, you should know that even a very small amount of alcohol consumed before bed can seriously affect sleep quality.[29] If you're not sleeping well, go to www.abigail-hardinphd.com for a separate, comprehensive guide to sleeping better.

Manage chronic stress

This is easier said than done. "Right, I'll just go ahead and remove all the stressors from my life during one of the worst economic and social upheavals in recent history in the midst of a global pandemic!" said no one, ever.

Let's be honest, these are extremely stressful times. It is important to recognize that you cannot self-care your way out of stress related to large-scale, systemic social and cultural issues like racism, inequality, bias, food insecurity, or other major life stressors. That being said, there are certainly small changes you can make yourself to help manage stress and limit how dramatically it influences your body and immune function. I recommend that if you have major life stress right now, that you seek therapy from a psychologist or another mental health expert. Why? *Therapy interventions, especially a type of therapy called Cognitive Behavioral Therapy (CBT) have been shown across multiple studies to improve immune function.*[30] If you don't want to do therapy, or if you don't have access to therapy due to a lack of insurance or other reasons, you can try some of the following stress management tips:

- ***Try meditating.*** Search online for free guided meditation videos or download an app to help you meditate. I personally use a meditation app called *Calm*, and it works well for me. I have good friends who swear by the app *Headspace.* Neither of these apps are free, but both have free trials available, at the time of writing. For a longer list of relaxation strategies, apps and techniques, go to my website, www.abigailhardinphd.com.
- ***Use deep breathing.*** While seated comfortably, place one hand on your belly and one hand on your chest. Notice which hand is moving more to determine if you are breathing shallowly (hand on your chest moving more) or deeply (hand on your belly moving more). Then, see if you can deepen and slow your breathing so that your belly hand moves most while your chest hand stays relatively still.
- ***Vent to a friend.*** Friends aren't the same as a therapist, but

they are still a great resource. Set up a weekly phone call with a trusted friend or relative who cares about you. Trade off venting to each other. Ask your friend to avoid problem-solving for you, but just to give you a gentle, listening ear. Social support reduces your risk of illness by reducing inflammation in the body.[31]

- *Take real breaks.* If at all possible, when you have breaks during your workday, actually take them rather than eating at your desk. Take a quick walk around the block (with a mask), do a short meditation session, stretch, or do desk yoga (search it on the internet – it's fun!).
- *Have some fun.* Break up stressful days by injecting a little fun. Find a stand-up comedy to watch on your TV streaming service or take a break with cute animal photos on the internet. You could also try board game night with your family, or set up a video conference happy hour with friends (drinking moderately, of course!).

Get safe, socially distanced exercise

Moderate exercise clearly improves immune function.[32] The CDC recommends adults get at least 150 minutes of moderate exercise, like brisk walking, per week.[33] But during the pandemic, it's important that this exercise conform to infection-prevention standards. Wearing a mask and socially distancing yourself from others is still critical. Consider going for a walk, jog, or wheelchair roll outside, making sure you can maintain six feet of distance from others. You might also consider going to parks, hiking, renting a kayak, etc.

You may recall that in Chapter 1, I noted that obesity is a risk factor for severe COVID-19 infection and death. In this chapter, I've covered eating nutritious foods and exercising, but I've included nothing about losing weight. If obesity is a risk factor for COVID-19, why not attempt to lose weight now? The reason is because there is overwhelming evidence that attempts to lose weight generally do not result in actual, sustained weight loss for most people, and at worst, can cause serious health problems like "yo-yo dieting" and eating disorders.[34,35]

Instead, think about weight as secondary to healthy habits. Healthy habits like eating well and exercising make a difference in your health and immunity, and a reduction in weight is a nice side-effect. If you're eating well, exercising regularly and avoiding frequent over-indulging, you may see some weight drop off naturally, depending on your physiology. However, if you focus on the outcome of losing weight, you may temporarily drop a few pounds, but depending on what you did to lose weight, you may risk harming your psychological and physical health.[36] Focus on eating well and taking care of yourself using the above strategies. Weight is not a good proxy for health; focus on behaviors, not the scale.

One last note before we move on – I don't recommend that you try to totally overhaul all your health behaviors all at once. That's a recipe for getting overwhelmed, feeling frustrated, and giving up. Use the self-evaluation of health behaviors chart available at www.abigailhardinphd.com to assess your current habits and to figure out what health habit could use your attention. Make small, sustainable changes only, and address one habit at a time.

Locate your nearest testing sites

Next, it's important to consider what steps you might take if you have been exposed to someone with COVID-19 or think you may have it but aren't sick enough to need emergency care. Consider looking into what options are available in order to get in touch with your primary care physician or local urgent care facility via telephone or video chat. Also, create a list of your nearest urgent care facilities, testing sites, pharmacies, or other places where you could get a test. Testing sites may change frequently, so I recommend you update this list every three weeks or so. If you work in the healthcare industry, find out what your employer's testing recommendations are and whether you can access testing through your work. Some employers may offer testing on-site or cover COVID-19 testing costs, preventing you from needing to find a testing site or pay out of pocket. Some insurance providers may also provide testing at low or no cost.

Research hospitals and care centers

Finally, in case you do ultimately need to go to the hospital, start researching the hospitals in your area and what quality of care they seem to provide. You can look at online rankings, ask friends about their hospital experiences, or call healthcare professionals you know. Check with your insurance provider about which hospitals are covered in your network, and which are not. Some insurance providers will cover multiple hospitals, and others will only cover one local hospital. Be sure to check if the hospital you choose to go to will have rehabilitation in-house, and therapies available to you even before you

emergency warning signs listed at the end of this chapter, you can begin by monitoring and treating your symptoms at home.

"If you start feeling symptoms, try not to panic. At the time we had it, it seemed like death was almost assured. Now we know that there is a good chance for recovery. Panic makes the symptoms feel worse."
- Matt

The first thing to do is to start tracking your symptoms. Get a piece of paper and log the dates and times of your symptoms. You should also start monitoring your temperature with a body thermometer at least once in the morning, afternoon and night. Write down your body temperatures.

"Keep symptom logs or a journal of some sort so that you can have that on hand for medical professionals."
– Kerri

"For someone who gets sick, please focus on rest and recovery. I think people should log their symptoms, in a systematic way, not so much as an obsession that can lead to unnecessary anxiety but in a way that can help medical professionals and other people understand the disease effects."
– Ray

In addition to tracking your symptoms, it is also recommended that you get a test for COVID-19. If you prepared a list of testing locations, you're already prepared. Otherwise, reach out to your primary care physician online or over the phone and tell them what you're experiencing. Then, get tested if they recommend, and follow the advice of your physician to manage symptoms at home. If symptoms get worse, call your physician back and update them. In terms of managing the symptoms themselves, there isn't a lot you can do at home to manage symptoms, except the basics you would do any other time you were feeling under the weather. According to the Mayo Clinic, you can try:[38]

- Getting plenty of rest
- Drinking plenty of fluids
- Taking over-the-counter pain relievers

Supporting your immune system while sick

If you're sick, there are a few things you can do to promote your immune system, and several things to avoid to ensure your immune system can fight for you. First, let me tell you a little about the human body's response to infections.

When humans are sick, they fall into a pattern of predictable behaviors called "sick behaviors."[39] Sick behaviors are adaptive, automatic behavioral responses that promote rest, sleep, and withdrawal from social environments. These behaviors are adaptive because they force the infected person to rest and withdraw from social environments, which may have the added benefit of reducing transmission of an infectious pathogen to others. Supporting your body while you're sick mostly involves allowing your sick behaviors to drive your recovery, and doing the things your mom taught you as a child: get plenty of rest, drink hot liquids/soup, and avoid socializing and alcohol.

If you're sick, respect your own body's sick behaviors. Make sure you get plenty of rest, and don't be tempted to stay up all night going down an internet hole about COVID-19, no matter how tempting. Getting enough rest when you're sick can help support your immune system as it fights off illness.[40]

Additionally, you may have heard the folk advice to "feed a cold and starve a fever". In credit to the wisdom of folk traditions, there is scientific evidence that there are different immune responses to feeding vs. fasting,[41] However it's not clear which approach may work best with COVID-19 infections. If you are sick but still have an appetite, reach for nutritious, balanced meals. Chicken soup might be a good option, since it has been demonstrated to effectively thin nasal mucous, assisting with clearance of upper respiratory infections.[42]

Finally, get plenty of hydration and avoid alcohol. Alcohol can interfere with your immune system's ability to fight off an infection.[43] Additionally, alcohol is dehydrating, and staying hydrated is an important component of managing respiratory infections.[44] However, if you are drinking lots of fluids, be sure to also replace your electrolytes – you can find electrolyte replacement drinks at your local drug store. Electrolytes are minerals found in your body that have an electric charge, like sodium, calcium and potassium. Electrolyte drinks can be unpleasant tasting unless they have added flavors and sugars, but try to find an electrolyte drink with as little sugar as possible.

When to go to the hospital

"The little of the news I watched was also scary, because you would hear about people who didn't go the hospital and died in their bed at night. Trying to figure when I was "really bad" that I would need more care was what really made me nervous."
- Hillary

As you manage your symptoms and support your immune system using the above strategies, it may be difficult to know if or when to go to the hospital. According to the Centers for Disease Control and Prevention (CDC), if you think you might have COVID-19, you should stay home and isolate yourself away from friends, family or visitors.[16] But, the World Health Organization specifically points out that anyone with severe symptoms, or with mild symptoms but risk factors for poor outcomes (older people or anyone with an underlying health condition) should be treated within a hospital.[45] If you have mild symptoms, call your primary care physician, get tested, and follow the advice of your physician. As long as your symptoms are mild, you can manage them at home. If you are at high risk, your physician may suggest you go to the hospital even if your symptoms are mild to moderate. However, if you are having any of the life-threatening symptoms listed below, go straight to the hospital or call 9-1-1.

You should recognize the following as warning signs of an emergency, and call 9-1-1 or go directly to an emergency room if you have any of the following:[46]

Hand this card over to your decision-maker when you are hospitalized. This will allow them to continue to pay bills and keep the household running while you're in the hospital. If you'd rather not create an index card with this information, you can store your login information and passwords in a safe at home and ensure someone you trust has access to the safe.

Other things that might be nice to have in your kit:

- *A caregiver for your children and activities to keep them busy. This can include crayons and coloring pages, a small soft toy, or a book.* If you go to the hospital and must bring children along with you, make sure you bring another trusted adult who can safely provide them with care once you're admitted. Keep them occupied with quiet, distracting games and activities. It doesn't hurt to include some crossword puzzle books, magazines, novels, etc. for yourself too. If you're feeling well enough to sit up and use these things, you will be glad you have them.

- *An inexpensive blanket (don't include grandma's heirloom quilt).* Hospitals have plenty of linens and blankets, but patients say that they feel much less anxious when they have something from home to touch. Don't bring anything expensive, or anything you would be upset about losing/getting soiled.

- *A small zip-close cosmetic bag or quart-sized plastic zip bag.* If you are being admitted to the hospital, use this bag to collect any important objects for your family to take home. Take off wedding rings, watches, jewelry, etc. and send them home with your family. Put your wallet in this bag as well. You may move around from room to room in the hospital, and small items can get lost in the shuffle.

If you have family taking you to the hospital, expect to be separated from them for infection control purposes. Also, be aware that once you are admitted, the hospital may not allow visitors, or seriously restrict visiting hours. Make sure you send healthy family members home with any important personal items for safekeeping. Hospitals usually have a safe, but it's best to keep your important rings, heirlooms, etc. at home. This is why I recommend bringing an old set of glasses or hearing aids. Small items like these can easily get misplaced or damaged in all the chaos of being in the hospital.

Your healthcare team

Typically, your team in the hospital will be led by a physician (someone with a doctoral-level medical degree) who coordinates a team roughly the size of an NFL game-day roster. The lead physician will be called your "attending physician" and if you are at a teaching hospital that is affiliated with a university, you will also have "fellow physicians", "resident physicians" and "interns" who are all physicians at various levels of training. Moreover, you may have "consulting physicians" or "consulting providers" who are not technically a member of your main medical team, but who are consulted to work with you because they have specialized knowledge your team thinks could benefit you.

You may also have advanced practice providers (APPs) on your team, like nurse practitioners and physician assistants. APPs can prescribe medications and order tests, just like the physicians.

While in the hospital you may also have a mental health expert working with you, like a psychologist, psychiatrist, or both. This person will help you manage changes in thinking and emotions that often come along with being ill. The hospital may also have a chaplain to attend to spiritual needs.

Each day, you will have a nurse and a patient care technician (PCT) who are responsible for your minute-to-minute needs like administering treatments and medications, bringing you items you need, helping you move around or reposition, etc. Your team will also include a social worker or case manager who is responsible for helping you and your family plan for a safe discharge from the hospital.

If you have difficulty breathing or require ventilation, you may have a respiratory therapist who monitors and adjusts settings on the machine. Other people you may encounter include a registered dietician to help identify a safe a nutritious menu for you, cleaning staff who ensure your room is sanitized regularly if it is safe for them to enter, and food service staff who help you order meals and bring them to you.

Finally, there will likely be a team of therapists who help you recover, including a physical therapist, an occupational therapist and a speech-language pathologist.

That is a very long list of people, and it will be hard to keep them all straight. Ask providers to write their names on the whiteboard in your room or keep pen and paper handy and write down the names and responsibilities of everyone who visits you. Keep in mind that if you have COVID-19, not everyone who is working for you may visit you in your room, in order to reduce the risk of infection for others in the hospital.

Rest assured even if you haven't seen a soul, you have a large team of very committed healthcare professionals working for you behind the scenes.

What will the hospital do for you?

One of the problems with COVID-19 is that it appears to cause a severe lung problem called acute respiratory distress syndrome, or ARDS.[47] ARDS can cause the lungs to fail, resulting in a condition called "hypoxemic respiratory failure", which essentially means not getting enough oxygen into the body and brain because of lung failure.

If you have ARDS, you can be treated with what's called "non-invasive ventilation" which includes oxygen through a mask or tubes in your nose. Or, you might have "invasive mechanical ventilation," in which a breathing tube is placed into the mouth and down the windpipe. You might also hear this referred to as "intubation." In some cases, the tube may be placed directly in through the neck, also known as a "tracheotomy".

In some cases, you may go through a process called "prone positioning", in which you are flipped onto your stomach periodically to reduce the work the lungs must do. Prone positioning helps by changing the air pressures in your lungs, improving how much blood can flow into your lungs, and lets the lungs expand easier because your chest and heart aren't pressing down on your lungs.[48] Prone positioning can be helpful but can also result in breakdown of the skin if you're in that position too long or too frequently. So, some survivors end up with wounds on their skin, possibly on their face where their face made contact with the pillow.

In addition to ensuring your lungs get the oxygen they need

via non-invasive or mechanical ventilation, the healthcare team may also support your body in fighting any bacterial infections that might take hold by providing antibiotics. And, to keep your body fluid levels normal, the team might also give fluids through a vein.[47]

Finally, if these medical strategies don't work, a last-resort option for treatment is extracorporeal membrane oxygenation, or ECMO.[47] ECMO works as a replacement lung outside the body. It pumps blood to the machine where the blood is filled with oxygen, and then pumps the oxygen-filled blood back into the body.[49]

If you become critically ill and require mechanical ventilation, invasive procedures or ECMO, you will be kept comfortable with sedating medications.[49] If this all sounds very scary, know that you are unlikely to remember many of these procedures due to the sedating medications that are designed to keep you calm and mostly unconscious.

How to get the best care from providers

In the past several years, I have seen families, patients and healthcare teams come together to become dream teams that produce amazing results. I've also seen what can only be described as "hurricanes of dysfunction" rip through families as they try, fruitlessly, to navigate communicating with their healthcare team. You definitely want to be in the former category. So, how do you, as the patient, get the best care from your hospital team? As a family member, how can you ensure you're helping your loved one get the best treatment possible?

Advocating for yourself as the patient

If you are a patient in the hospital, especially if you're in a critical care unit (an ICU) or an acute unit (like the medical floor), please remember that the nurses and physicians you see are in the business of saving lives. Your comfort and needs matter, and even your wants are important. But try to keep in mind that if you push your call light and no one comes, it could be because they were helping someone who was in critical need of lifesaving care in that moment. Hospital staff are well trained to know what is an emergency and what isn't, and they prioritize accordingly. So, if you request help but your need isn't being prioritized, it is because staff are assisting someone else who desperately needs help in that moment. By waiting patiently, you are helping someone else efficiently receive lifesaving care. See if you can think about being in the hospital as an opportunity to feel connected to your fellow patients. If you take the perspective of "we're all in this together" you'll find it's easier to tolerate the moments of frustration when you have to wait.

That being said, sometimes it can still be extremely frustrating to feel as though you're reliant on someone else, who may not always come immediately to help when you need or want it.

Below are some tricks you can use to get the best possible care from your providers:

- *Lump your requests into single visits.* For instance, if you think you may need a glass of water, a bedpan, some pain medication and for someone to help you reach the TV

- **Stay grounded.** Stress affects us all differently. If you are the kind of person who gets angry when you're stressed, make sure you take the space you need to prevent lashing out. If you're visiting in the hospital and something goes wrong, you may feel upset at the team, or at the hospital itself. If this happens, take some time to go for a walk. Your feelings are totally valid. But, if you lash out at staff by threatening them, becoming violent or using offensive language, you can risk being prevented from visiting again. Once you're feeling calm, if you'd like, you can ask for the customer service or "patient experience" phone number and make a report.

Supporting your loved one (even if you can't be by their side)

Being a family member of someone with COVID-19 and not being able to be with them during their hospitalization can be heart-wrenching. It feels so isolating to be on the outside looking in, waiting for news from the healthcare team. But just because you can't be there doesn't mean you can't help.

Here are some suggestions for how to help, even when you can't be by their side:

- **Quickly identify whether your loved one might be having delirium.** Delirium is a change in your thinking and/or your perception that comes on suddenly and then might fluctuate over time.[50] See Chapter 5 for more details on the types of delirium and how to recognize them. If your loved one is awake enough to take phone calls, call regularly

(I usually recommend 3 times per day). If you suspect they may be experiencing delirium, use the phone call to re-orient them. Say something like "Hey honey, it's your wife/husband. It's about 3pm on Friday, August 17th, and I'm calling you while you're in the hospital to say I love you and to hang in there." I know this kind of a call sounds weird, but keeping your loved one oriented to you, their location, the time and the date will help their brain stay grounded through all the daunting delirium symptoms. You can also provide reassurance by saying "I can't be there because of the visitor restrictions, but I want you to know I've been thinking about you all day. I'm gathering up all your favorite recipes so we can have your favorite meal when you finally come home. You can do this!" You should also know that delirium can cause rapidly fluctuating emotions, causing people to lash out or act differently. If you observe this, stay calm, offer your loved one reassurance, and let the healthcare team know.

- *Bring in photos.* You can bring in large-format photos or posters of your family, pets, favorite memories, etc. These can help with orientation, reduce anxiety, and be a reminder of all the support they have at home. You can also bring in favorite items like blankets or pillows, if the nurse says it's OK.
- *Make reassuring posters and have everyone in your family sign them.* Phrases like "Keep Fighting – We Believe In You!" and "We Love You – Stay Positive!" may seem silly at a time like this. But as a healthcare provider myself, I have personally had COVID-19 survivors tell me that posters like these from family were the reason they felt they were able to hang on, keep fighting and survive.

Caring for children when a parent tests positive

Depending on how old your kids are, their reaction to a parent being sick or hospitalized can be different. Some children may not even understand what an illness or a hospital is. Others may have a very good idea about COVID-19 and how dangerous it can be.

> *"The hardest part of all was having to be away from my six-year-old son while in isolation, he did not know why he could only talk to me over the balcony or why he could not give me hugs. He did in an abstract way, but this was all new to him."*
> - Danielle

For very young children (pre-school or younger), having a parent in the hospital can be confusing and anxiety-provoking. It is possible they will think that something they've done, thought or believed caused the parent to become sick. It's important to reassure them that while lots of kids might think like this, it's not true.[52] They might worry that they will also get sick. Because children don't fully understand bodies and illness, it is important to answer their questions with honest, accurate information. But it is also important to make sure the information is simplified for them. Using picture books that show anatomy can help. There is a list of children's books and resources you might find useful at www.abigailhardinphd.com. Also, use very simple phrases, like "Mom has a sickness in her lungs, and the doctors and nurses are keeping it from getting worse." At this age, give children a "job" to do to help, even if they can't come to the hospital to visit. You might have them

56

make posters, cards, or drawings for the family member's room. Help them add entries to the ICU diary, which is explained in Chapter 5.

For school-age children, their worries might be easier to say out loud. They may reasonably have fears about catching COVID-19. Try to reassure children this age with simple but truthful language, like, "The nurses and doctors have seen many people with this illness who have gotten better." Involve children this age in making posters, cards and drawings. Have them write in the ICU diary.

Adolescents and older children should be able to talk about their thoughts and feelings but may not want to. Try to respect their privacy while also making sure your child knows that it's OK to express what they're going through. You can demonstrate sharing emotions by saying something like "You know, today I was feeling really nervous about grandpa being in the hospital. I had to remind myself that he is being cared for by a team of experts before I could feel better." You can also try asking "What's your understanding of what's going on right now?" or "How are you feeling about dad being in the hospital?" Because they're old enough to understand, clear and accurate information should always be provided to adolescents. Adolescents can participate in making cards and posters, if they want. However, they may prefer to do something privately, like writing a song or poem, journaling, or texting/calling their friends.

If it comes time to have your children visit the hospital, you should reach out to the team and request a consultation with a type of provider called a child life specialist. This specialist can help prepare your children to visit the hospital, especially if they will see confusing or concerning medical devices or equipment. Although most children will not be able to see a hospitalized parent with an active COVID-19 infection, visiting later on during rehabilitation or another time when the family member has a negative COVID-19 test might be possible. If you plan to take your children to the hospital for a visit, prepare them with an idea of what you'll do during the visit. Give them a specific task or tasks to do, like hanging up a picture, telling a story, or showing pictures of something fun they did recently.[52]

Sometimes families are tempted to keep information away from children because they're worried about scaring them. Remember, children can pick up on even very small changes in their environment and in the behaviors of the adults around them. Do not lie to your children. Do respond honestly to any questions they have. At the same time, it's important not to use a child as someone to "vent" to, or to alarm them with excessive details that they haven't asked about. Be sure that you as the parent have another adult to talk to for support.

Being hospitalized can be uncomfortable and stressful, both for the patient and family. If you are prepared for hospitalization and make the most of it by following the above suggestions, you are doing everything you can to help yourself heal. In the next chapter, I'll cover what to expect if you become critically ill. Critical illness can be particularly frightening, so this would be a good time to take a self-care break if you feel like it. The next chapters are here for you when you're ready.

5

If You Become Critically Ill

"When I woke up, I felt like I had an elephant sitting on my chest...I was pretty loopy. I wanted my phone; they gave it to me, but I had forgotten how to use it. As the days went by, I was still a little loopy but getting better. My sister called; I really couldn't talk but I could listen. She tells me that I had been put into a drug induced coma. I had been given paralyzing meds to stop me from yanking out tubes. While I was under all of my organs shut down on me if they put me in the wrong position. I suffered acute renal [kidney] failure, double pneumonia, acute hypoxemia [low blood oxygen], it went after my heart and liver. I had to learn how to walk again (lost 40% of my muscle mass). I couldn't even swallow right anymore.

When I was finally able to go home, I was assigned a physical therapist, etc. I was terrified to go to sleep because I was reliving all the hallucinations I dreamt

*while in the coma. They were so real that to this day I
don't know what was real and what wasn't."*
- Stacie

Depending on how ill you are when you go to the hospital, you may go to a medical floor, or to an intensive care unit (ICU) directly. If you are sick enough to need the supervision of nurses and physicians, you'll go to a medical floor. If you're so sick you require lifesaving and critical care, you'll go to the ICU. Sometimes, if you are on a medical floor but something changes, like you start breathing poorly, you may be moved to an ICU to get a higher level of care. Once you're doing better, you may move back to the medical floor.

There are some things you should know about being critically ill with COVID-19. You may have symptoms aside from those mentioned in Chapter 1 of this book, especially if you are in critical condition. The following sections discuss some of the common problems associated with being critically ill, and what you can do to help even while you're still in the hospital.

Earlier, I talked about some of the more extreme lifesaving measures you might receive if you are critically ill, like receiving mechanical ventilation or being placed on ECMO. The good news is that if your COVID-19 infection results in you needing to be mechanically ventilated or placed on ECMO support, the healthcare team will keep you comfortable with sedating medications that keep you calm, still, and unconscious as necessary. Thus, it's possible that if you become critically ill, you won't remember parts or all of your critical illness due to the illness and the effects of these medications.

Although being critically ill is very frightening, by simply reading this book you are mentally preparing in ways that will help you recover if you do get very sick. You may have heard the phrase "it's never too late to begin" and that same thinking applies for COVID-19. By reading this you are preparing yourself mentally for the possibility of a critical illness, and in doing so setting the tone now for your recovery. You should know that the path your recovery will take starts in the ICU. As soon as you are alert and awake, you begin setting the tone for how you will recover.

Post-Intensive Care Syndrome

As you awaken from sedation, you may notice symptoms that weren't there at first. This is because as your body fights the virus, your body's immune system can overreact, causing damage.[53] Additionally, the treatments provided to people with COVID-19 can cause their own side effects.[54] There is a set of symptoms that people with severe illnesses of any kind (not just COVID-19) commonly experience, called "Post Intensive Care Syndrome", or PICS.[55] Over 50% of people who have been in the ICU develop at least some symptoms of PICS.[56] PICS is seen in lots of critical illnesses, and is likely to be seen in those with severe COVID-19 infections.[57]

So, what is PICS? PICS is a syndrome, meaning it is a bunch of symptoms that seem to all hang together, but isn't necessarily its own disease. Symptoms of PICS include:

- Body weakness
- Thinking changes

- Emotional changes

I'll go into each of these symptoms, and how best to handle them.

Body Weakness

Being in the ICU can very quickly result in incapacitating weakness. In less than a week, muscles can begin to waste away as you lie on the bed without moving.[58] In addition to muscles wasting away, lying in bed can cause damage to nerves, making it hard to move muscles, even if the muscles are still there.[18] Muscles related to swallowing can also be affected, making it unsafe to swallow foods or liquids, also known as "dysphagia."[59]

Early mobilization, even before you leave the ICU, is the key to starting to gain back strength. In fact, early mobilization can begin before you're even off a ventilator, if you were placed on one.[56] We normally think of physical therapy (PT) and occupational therapy (OT) as things we do after we're no longer sick, but in fact PT and OT are often available in the ICU and most other floors in the hospital. This is one of the reasons why I recommend you research hospitals and the availability of rehabilitation in advance.

When early mobilization does happen, people leave the ICU much stronger, and sometimes faster, than those who didn't mobilize.[56] If you are awake, request PT and OT and participate as soon as possible. If you are not awake, a family member should ask to have you mobilized as soon as possible. Early mobilization might not always be possible, depending on whether you are still positive for COVID-19, because of infection control policies. But ask anyway.

Thinking Changes

PICS can result in thinking changes, also known as cognitive changes, or "delirium". Some might also use the term "encephalopathy". In essence, all these words and phrases mean the same thing: you're not thinking as clearly as you were before. Some people describe PICS thinking changes as feeling "foggy" or "out of it." Healthcare providers will usually use the term "delirium." Thinking changes can impact how you pay attention, how well you remember, your ability to organize your thoughts clearly and logically, and even how you navigate around or perceive things you see.

Delirium is a change in your thinking and/or your perception that comes on suddenly and then might fluctuate over time.[50] Scientists usually break delirium into two groups, based on the main symptoms. These are hypoactive delirium, and hyperactive delirium, explained here:[50]

Hypoactive Delirium

- Is very common but is less obvious to see than hyperactive delirium
- People seem withdrawn and lethargic
- Decreased movement and responsiveness/sluggishness
- Lack of motivation to do anything
- Lack of emotional expressions or facial expressions

Hyperactive Delirium

- Less common but very easy to see
- Agitation and restlessness
- Seeing or hearing things that aren't there (hallucinations)
- Believing things that aren't true (delusions)
- Might result in people being uncooperative and pulling out their tubes or medication lines

Not only is delirium a problem generally for people in the ICU, but with COVID-19 specifically, the chances of having delirium might be even higher. If you're in the ICU with COVID-19, you may have less access and connection to your family and fewer opportunities for delirium interventions from staff as they try to limit their exposure to you while you're still contagious. This isolation can result in disorientation that makes delirium more likely and more severe.[60] Not only that, but because COVID-19 may require you to be placed on your stomach for "prone positioning", the dosages of sedatives you require to keep you comfortable might be higher. So, the risk of delirium goes up due to the higher dosages of sedatives.[60]

> *"The scariest part was being delusional. I made a post on Facebook that sounded like I was coming to terms with dying. 12 days isolation in the hospital took a toll on my mental health. My biggest concern is that I may never recover."*
> - Mindy

The problem with delirium is that the longer it goes on, the more likely you are to have difficulty getting back into your daily life and the more likely you are to be disabled nearly a year later.[61] That's why it's so important to catch it, and treat it, early.

Another concern is that although delirium is generally reversible, some thinking problems can last long-term. Thinking clearly after an ICU stay may be even harder if you had ARDS, the respiratory failure syndrome that COVID-19 causes. Studies of long-term thinking problems after ARDS from diseases other than COVID-19 report that 70% of recovered patients had significant thinking problems at the time of hospital discharge, 45% still had problems with their thinking a year later, and 47% still had problems two years later, possibly due to reduced oxygen to the brain.[62]

Unfortunately, even though many people receive rehabilitation therapies after being critically ill, cognitive testing is not common – only about 12% of people are ever tested to see if their thinking skills have changed.[62] You will read in Chapter 7 that it is important you select a rehabilitation facility that will have the necessary experts to diagnose and treat any cognitive changes you experience as a result of your COVID-19 infection and PICS.

Delirium is more likely to happen during your ICU stay if you have a history of heavy alcohol use, have a history of high blood pressure, or if you receive heavy doses of sedating drugs during your ICU stay.[18] This means that during the COVID-19 pandemic, it would be wise to avoid excessive alcohol use, and be sure to continue to take blood pressure medications, exercise, and eat nutritious food if you can. If you need a reminder on healthy habits to change now, you can flip back to Chapter 2.

The faster you can identify that you have delirium, the faster you can start to reverse it. Because of these reasons, it is very important that delirium or other thinking changes are identified and treated while you're in the hospital. Family members can help a loved one in the ICU with cognitive changes by taking these steps:

- *Ask the team to assess your loved one for delirium.* Do this especially if they seem more sluggish, less responsive, or aren't showing their normal emotions/facial expressions.
- *Ask the team what they do for management of delirium.* Check to make sure they're keeping sedation at a minimum, if possible.
- *Stay connected.* Stay in contact with family, friends, clergy, or other support systems as much as possible. If your loved one is sedated in the ICU, ask to see if you can still talk to them over the phone, even if they can't respond to you.
- *Reorient your loved one.* If you can connect with your loved one in the ICU, try to help them stay oriented by explaining to them where they are, where you are, why they're in the hospital, and reassure them about all the care they're receiving in order to get better. If your loved one had glasses or hearing aids in their COVID-19 kit, ask the nurse to help your loved one wear them daily, so they can stay connected to the world around them through all senses.
- *Be a cheerleader.* If the nurse will let you, drop off posters, big photographs, or signs to put up in the room that say things like "We love you Mom" or "You can do this – Beat COVID!" – whatever you think your loved one would find helpful.
- *Request early mobilization with PT and OT.* Starting the

rehabilitation process early is the key to getting stronger even before leaving the ICU.

- ***Request cognitive evaluation.*** Request that the team consult a speech-language pathologist or a rehabilitation psychologist/neuropsychologist as early as possible.

Emotional Changes

PICS can also cause emotional changes, like symptoms of depression, anxiety, or other conditions like post-traumatic stress disorder (PTSD).[63] Even three months after leaving the hospital, 37% of people who were in an ICU still experience at least mild depression. That number only drops to 33% even a full year after discharge. And seven percent of people still have symptoms of PTSD a year after they discharge.[63]

But here's the problem: while the U.S. healthcare system is pretty good at saving lives, it is pretty terrible at adequately addressing emotional concerns. Depending on where you live and what hospital you go to, you might not have a mental health professional available to you who is trained to treat emotional changes that result from critical illness. In fact, you might not have access to any mental health professional at all. There are a variety of reasons for this very serious oversight in our healthcare system, but that is a topic for another book altogether. Suffice it to say, if you are at a hospital with mental health care available, take full advantage of it. But there is a chance you won't be able to get the care you need, so you may need to rely on other sources of support.

"Right now, I'm seeing a therapist to help me learn to cope with it all. For a long time, I thought I was going

crazy because I couldn't sleep, I would have horrible nightmares and hallucinations from reliving the dreams I suffered while in the drug-induced coma. I also suffer from 'survivor's guilt'; the gentleman I got it from passed away."
- Stacie

Ask your team if there is a psychologist you can work with while you're in the hospital if you notice depression or anxiety. If there is no psychologist available, ask to speak to your social worker, or a psychiatrist. A chaplain might also be available for support, if spirituality is important to you. Also, don't forget that you can get support outside the hospital. Use your cell phone to call or video chat with your loved ones, a pastor, or friends. If you don't have one or don't know how to video chat, ask your nurse to help you. Tell people how you are feeling and what kind of support you need. If you already had a therapist before you were sick, reach out to them and ask for resources.

Remember, even if you are not normally the kind of person to talk about your emotions, these are unusual circumstances. Treat the emotional symptoms of PICS just like you would any other health symptom: talk to your healthcare team about them and make sure they are taken seriously and treated. After you leave the hospital, plan on working with a psychologist to manage your emotional changes in outpatient visits. Don't just go on suffering without telling anyone. Your symptoms do not mean you are deficient or not strong enough. They are common and treatable.

Finally, PICS isn't the only potential problem related to COVID-19 survival. As most critical care healthcare professionals know, PICS is something that affects survivors of critical illness in general. But there may also be long-term symptoms unique to COVID-19 that trouble survivors well after they test negative. At the time of writing this book, symptoms related to PICS and symptoms related to other long-term problems from COVID-19 aren't well enough understood for me to write much about it. But, anecdotally, individual survivors of COVID-19 complain of things like hair loss, pain, insomnia, fatigue, breathlessness and other symptoms months after their recovery. Future researchers will need to use large-scale studies to learn more about the aftermath of COVID-19.

Keeping a COVID-19 Diary

If your loved one spends significant time in the ICU with a breathing machine, or has to be sedated to be kept comfortable, it is likely that they will have some trouble remembering some parts or even all of their ICU stay. This is totally normal, but can be unnerving when they realize later they are missing memories. An extremely important, and often overlooked, task that you can do for your loved one with COVID-19 is to keep a COVID-19 diary.

The COVID-19 diary helps to keep track of the important daily events of the hospitalization. It works like this: the loved ones of someone critically ill in the hospital keep a diary to track the important day-to-day events that the person who's critically ill might not remember or might not remember well. If your loved one is isolated in the ICU, you may not be there to keep track of everything, but you can use the information you get from phone calls with the nurses and physicians to add to the diary. Write down things like what type of tests or treatments your loved one had, what changes occurred, and what type of progress was made each day. Important milestones to record can include getting a test, being placed on or taken off a ventilator, getting or removing a feeding tube, opening their eyes, saying first words, taking first bites of food, etc. Don't worry about small things like exact medication dosages, what time things happened, etc. Write just like you're writing a letter to your loved one each day, using your normal everyday language and including things you think they would want to know later. You can also include things from outside of the hospital, like what is going on at home each day, news and events, how the kids are doing, etc. You can find a sample COVID-19 diary page with entries on my website, www.abigailhardinphd.com.

The important thing is that you have a diary of what happened during this time, so that later, when your loved one is feeling better, they can look back and "fill in the blanks" in their memory. Diaries like these can help people recover from severe illness with fewer mental health symptoms.[64] Humans tend to think of our lives as stories – it's a natural tendency we have. When we lose memories, it's like someone ripped a few chapters out of the middle of the story, and then later, the ending is hard to make sense of. By keeping this diary, you are safely storing those middle chapters for your loved one. Just like it's a lot easier to make sense of a book when you read the whole thing front to back, it's a lot easier to put together the "story" of yourself as a survivor if you have all the chapters.

By the way, some people might not want to read the diary once they feel better. They would rather leave their memories blank. That's OK. If you keep a diary and they don't use it, don't pressure them. It's all about having the option.

Leaving the ICU

So, what comes next? As your illness improves, the healthcare team may start encouraging you to do some early mobilization, if it is safe given the isolation policies in the hospital. After that, your team may start asking you and your family to consider hospital discharge options. There may be several discharge options, including going to another floor of the hospital to receive more care, transferring to another facility, or going home. One discharge option may be acute rehabilitation, which you can read more about in Chapter 7.

If you had any symptoms of PICS and you are working with the team to plan your discharge, be sure to consider not just your physical changes, but your emotions and thinking as well. If you are going to rehabilitation, choose a rehabilitation facility that has the staff necessary to address emotional and cognitive changes. For instance, if you had changes in thinking, ensure that you will have access to speech therapy, and also to a neuropsychologist or rehabilitation psychologist. Psychologists can evaluate thinking using sensitive tests that will accurately show the changes in your thinking. Then, you can work with your speech-language pathologist on cognitive rehabilitation.

Recovering from critical illness is an important turning point in the COVID-19 experience. It marks the transition away from a focus on pure, physiological survival needs, and toward survivorship, rehabilitation and restarting life. These topics are covered in detail in the following chapters.

6

Surviving COVID-19

At the opening of the book, I told you that survival is not the goal if you have COVID-19, just the starting point. The real goal is to be able to thrive after you survive. Survival is funny that way – we think it's the only thing we care about until we have it, and then we realize it wasn't the goal at all. In this chapter you will read about chances of survival, identifying yourself as a survivor, and thinking about your survivorship as actually being somewhere in the middle of your whole COVID-19 journey. If that all sounds a bit overwhelming, just know this book doesn't end here, just like your journey doesn't end here. Let's continue this journey together, hand in hand.

The high rate of survival

One small silver lining of the COVID-19 pandemic appears to be that the percentage of those who die from it appears relatively low, around 2%.[5] So, even if you do get infected, with good quality medical care and a little luck, you have a reasonable chance of survival.

However, if your illness becomes severe and you do enter the intensive care unit (ICU), there are some factors that you should know about that can influence the likelihood of survival.

Severe cases can be supported with mechanical ventilation, or if that fails, extracorporeal membrane oxygenation, or ECMO. But in some cases patients may arrive to the ICU too late for these interventions to be effective. Additionally, even with life-saving care, COVID-19 can result in organ failure or shock, resulting in death. The stress of COVID-19 on the body can exacerbate pre-existing conditions like heart disease.[65] And, importantly, the personnel, equipment and beds must be available for these interventions to work, which is why having hospitals overrun with cases results in more deaths.[66]

Up to this point in the book, if you have done the following things, you are already doing everything in your power to survive:

- Read the previous chapters on prevention and preparation
- Read and are using the strategies for keeping yourself safe
- Kept up with your health, medications and are eating and exercising well

If you are reading this as you continue your battle with COVID-19, turn back to the chapters on hospitalization and critical care. The next chapters will be waiting for you when it's time, finally, to focus on recovery.

Unlike a car crash or an earthquake, it may be difficult to know when to call yourself a "survivor" of COVID-19. In some cases, it might be quite apparent, for example if you are moved to a rehabilitation unit or facility and your team says that you are medically stable. But what if you never went to the hospital? If you're treating yourself at home, you may feel like a survivor once the most severe symptoms and fevers have stopped. Continue to track your symptoms and body temperature and keep in contact with your physician. Your physician can help you keep tabs on the symptoms and work with you to identify when you have "turned the corner." Another way to know is to get another COVID-19 test once you are feeling better, which will tell you whether you still have an active COVID-19 infection.

Once you have decided you are indeed a survivor, then it's time to start focusing on your recovery. If you never went to the hospital and don't require rehabilitation, there may be a period of time while you are quarantined, or waiting for lingering symptoms to subside, when you can call yourself a survivor. At this time, you are still mostly resting, waiting for the next phase of healing to begin. If you find yourself in that state, I recommend you finish reading this chapter, then skip ahead to Chapter 8, where you will learn about getting back into your daily routine.

You have reached the top of the mountain!...

Maybe you're reading this while you and your family are healthy, but hoping to prepare, just in case. Maybe you're reading this in your hospital room, having been recently told that you're generally stable, and will be transitioning to another floor soon. Either way, I cannot stress enough the following two things, which are, weirdly enough, both true at the same time:

- If you have survived COVID-19, you should celebrate. You can be incredibly proud of yourself and your body for the amazing fight it put up. Congratulations!
- The fight does not stop here. Surviving COVID-19 is only the beginning of a new journey.

After you survive COVID-19, it is unlikely that the journey of recovery is over. It is more likely that you will have several more weeks, or even months, of recovery in front of you. The following chapters highlight some of the symptoms you might have, and how to manage them. The next chapters also introduce you to the idea of "rehabilitation" which is the process of gaining back the highest level of independence and function possible after a severe health event.

> *"I would want others to realize that COVID-19 recovery is different for everyone, my son had it and was OK in a week, I have been dealing with it for 5 months and a little better each month but still not myself at all. It can be frustrating and hard to explain to others that you do not feel like the same person you use to be before COVID-19. Emotionally and physically I am reminded of COVID-19 every day."*
> - Hillary

… And now you have to reach the next rock

Before we get into the next steps - rehabilitation, going home, and all that - I have a quick story for you. Stick with me. There is a method to my madness:

I was watching this really cool documentary movie called

Touching the Void (2003), and as a rehabilitation psychologist, I couldn't help but see the relevance to my patients. In the movie - which is based on true events - a mountain climber named Joe Simpson falls while climbing a really dangerous mountain peak in Peru. This next part contains spoilers – skip ahead if you want to watch the movie. Essentially, he falls into a large crevasse (a deep crack or fissure) and is assumed to be dead by his partner, who returns to base camp. All alone on the mountain, with frostbite, no supplies, and a broken leg, he must crawl - army-style - back to the base camp. Simpson recalls that the only way he was able to get down the mountain, without giving up, was by focusing on small goals along the way. He said that he felt overwhelmed and that he might give up when he thought about how much farther he still had to go down the mountain. But, when he told himself "I just need to get to that rock over there," he could make it. Then he set his sights on the next rock a few more feet away. Then the next one. Then the next one.

If you have survived the initial COVID-19 infection, you have just fallen into the crevasse and lived. Now, you need to climb down the mountain. Simpson could do it, and you can do it too. In fact, I know for a fact you can do it because I have personally watched countless other COVID-19 survivors make the same journey. Take Simpson's advice and try not to get overwhelmed by how much recovery you have in front of you. Do not get discouraged if your body seems slow to recover. Pick the "rock" that represents what you need to do today to recover, and just focus on getting there. Maybe you only focus on one thing, like doing a PT session. Do that one thing, then pick the next "rock", and so on and so forth.

By the way, Simpson survives the whole ordeal, makes it back to basecamp, and has a movie made about him. You can make it back to basecamp. Just keep crawling.

7

Rehabilitation

You have made it through the worst at this point. You are medically stable and now ready to do the hard work of getting stronger, more able, and clearer headed. Rehabilitation may not be easy, especially if you've been sick and hospitalized. You might feel frustrated that you still have so much recovery left in front of you. But remember this: you're coming down the side of the mountain; just focus on the one rock ahead of you, one at a time, and take your time. (Re-read the story in Chapter 6 if you need a refresher). And know you're not alone.

Rehabilitation literally means to "make able." It's the process of helping you achieve the highest level of function and independence that you can while improving your quality of life. Rehabilitation does not mean turning back the clock and making your body just as it was before you had COVID-19. There is still no medical intervention that can "undo" what's happened. But rehabilitation can help you get back to the things and people you love.

Before I go into the details of rehabilitation, I'll touch on some of the "long-haul" symptoms you might be now experiencing as a survivor.

Managing Long-Haul COVID-19 Symptoms

"I'm still on oxygen and breathing treatments. I am still extremely fatigued. Somedays all that gets done is a shower."
– Tammy

In Chapter 5, I outlined the symptoms of PICS (Post-Intensive Care Syndrome) and how to manage them while you're still in the ICU. Briefly, they include body weakness, changes in thinking and changes in emotions

"The brain fog is intense. I found myself pausing at work today because I went completely blank as to what I was doing..."
- Tia

"I am currently dealing with cognitive issues, neuropathy, [and] severe fatigue."
- Tati

There are also some other symptoms that you should know about, in addition to the symptoms of PICS. Because of the strong inflammatory (immune) response in your body during a severe COVID-19 infection, and possibly also due to a bacterial infection that took hold while your body was weak, you may have developed heart failure, liver failure, kidney failure or shock.[67] Work with your healthcare team to find out if damage was done to your organs, and if so, if it can be treated or reversed. Some people may need long-term kidney treatments like dialysis. After you leave the hospital, your healthcare team will refer you to medical specialists for any follow-up you will need (kidney doctors, liver doctors, heart doctors, etc.). You may also experience skin wounds. Being on your stomach in the process called "prone positioning" can help you survive COVID-19 but can also result in skin breakdown on your face or front. If you were on your back for a long time, you might have skin breakdown on your buttocks or elsewhere on your back. These wounds will need to be cared for so they can heal.

Continue to track your symptoms when you leave the hospital, and request referrals to specialists. Scientists still don't know everything there is to know about COVID-19, so it is hard to know exactly what symptoms might totally resolve, and what new ones might pop up. Also, because this disease is so new, it is possible you might be contacted by your local health department or research departments within the hospital where you were treated. If someone contacts you about your COVID-19 symptoms, be sure to verify their affiliation before sharing your private health information.

Rehabilitation

Rehabilitation generally happens in two different phases: In the first phase, called *acute rehabilitation,* you may spend time in a rehabilitation unit or special rehabilitation hospital. Your healthcare team will evaluate you in the hospital and make a recommendation about whether or not the acute form is necessary.

The second phase of rehabilitation happens after you leave

the hospital. Depending on your insurance coverage, your location, and what is medically appropriate for you, you might have rehabilitation therapies in your own home or outpatient appointments at a special rehabilitation clinic or center.

Depending on the severity of your COVID-19 symptoms and how you're functioning when you become medically stabilized, you may skip the first phase of rehabilitation and discharge from the hospital straight to your home, where you will begin the second-phase therapies.

If you were not hospitalized but find that you are having trouble returning to your previous level of physical, emotional, or cognitive functioning, you may need to contact your primary care physician to request an outpatient rehabilitation referral. This can include evaluation of your thinking and memory by a psychologist or speech-language pathologist.

Acute Rehabilitation

While you are in the hospital, you will be evaluated by a team of rehabilitation experts, including physicians and therapists, who can help you and your family decide if acute rehabilitation is the right move for you. If acute rehabilitation is a good fit, you will work with your healthcare team to initiate a referral to an acute rehabilitation unit or center. This first phase of rehabilitation is different from other parts of the hospitalization. In acute rehabilitation, you will need to complete three hours or more of daily therapies. These therapies are essentially workouts for your brain and body to help you achieve your highest level of independence possible. Acute rehabilitation is not designed for you to complete all your goals and get back to exactly how you functioned before. Rather, it's designed to get your body

this case, also call ahead to the various rehabilitation centers and make sure you will have access to all the professionals you need. Keep in mind that if you had delirium or other thinking changes, or emotional changes, you will want to make sure your rehabilitation center has a psychologist of some kind (a neuropsychologist or rehabilitation psychologist) and a speech-language pathologist.

Rehabilitation Timeline

Most people will stay in an acute rehabilitation unit for a few weeks. Some will stay only a few days, and less commonly, some will stay a month or more.

After you discharge from acute rehabilitation, expect to complete more therapies in the second phase as an outpatient, or in sessions at home. This phase generally lasts longer—months, rather than days. Instead of completing three hours of therapy a day, you may do three hours of therapy a week. This "low and slow" style of therapy will help you maximize your recovery while allowing your body the time it needs to do necessary repairs to strengthen itself.

Your rehabilitation coverage benefits may end for a number of reasons, including running out of benefits from your insurance, your healthcare team determining that you've reached the highest level of independence they can give you, or ideally, meeting your own goals.

Rehabilitation experiences vary

Your rehabilitation experience will be largely dependent on you and what you make of it. Many people find it exhausting and difficult to do three hours of therapy every day. That being said, if you view the therapies as getting you closer to your goals each day, even if they're tiring and difficult, you will stay motivated.

Use the "Rehabilitation Goals" worksheet available at www.abigailhardinphd.com to share with your rehabilitation team what personal goals you're working on. The worksheet will help you set your goals clearly, and help your team communicate to you how their therapies will get you the results you want

One thing you should know right off the bat is that not everyone will be able to go directly home from an acute rehabilitation program. Many patients go to another facility, where they can continue to heal, get stronger, and get therapies at a less-intense pace until they're ready to go home. These facilities may be called "Sub-Acute Rehabilitation" or "Skilled Nursing Facilities" depending on your region. Going to another facility after acute rehabilitation is often a very good idea. Don't see it as a failure. See it as getting to the next rock on your way to basecamp (home).

Reasons to go to another facility might include:

- There is no one at home who can provide the care you need, and it would be safer to have the staff available to you at a facility until you're able to function more independently.
- There is someone at home to help, but they can't be around

throughout the day when you need care, for instance, if they are working a full-time job.

- The home environment is too difficult to get around in, especially if you will be using a walker, wheelchair, or cane.
- It feels safer to you or your family to have nursing providing full-time nursing care for your loved one, rather than taking it over yourselves.

Talk to the rehabilitation team as early as possible about where you want to go after you discharge, and what you and they think is realistic. Remember, taking things one step at a time is safe, and might be the best fit for you and your family.

Making the most of your acute rehabilitation

One mistake I see a lot in rehabilitation is that people assume they will be able to get through three hours a day of therapy without preparing themselves physically and mentally. The truth is, three hours a day of therapies may not sound like a lot, but when you're doing it, it feels like bootcamp. In order to reach your goals, you'll need to give 100% in therapies. In order to give 100%, your brain and body need to be fueled and rested.

Here are some tips for making the most of your therapies:

- *Before each therapy session, think to yourself what your biggest goals are.* Say to yourself, "I'm doing this session so that I can [insert your goal here: walk, cook for my family, etc.]"
- *Tell your therapists what you need stay motivated.* For

instance, if you're trying to walk without a walker, but you're afraid you might fall, tell your therapists about your fear so that they can help you by standing behind you with a chair, or holding you up with a strap.

- *Go to bed on time.* Hospital life starts early – like around 5:00AM. Try to be in bed, with lights out, no later than 9:30PM. Shut the TV and phone off at least 30 minutes before you hope to fall asleep to give your brain some time to wind down.

- *Tell your team if you can't sleep.* They can help with medications or relaxation strategies. Sometimes they might even have earplugs, sleep masks, decaffeinated tea, or other sleep aides you can try.

- *Talk to your friends and family about how you're doing.* I have worked directly with marines, firefighters, and other "guy's guys" who tell me that expressing their feelings to loved ones or a psychologist was critical to success in rehabilitation. Getting your feelings out means you have more mental space and energy to focus on your therapies and getting stronger.

- *Eat.* Ask your team about any special diets you're on. Try to eat as much of each meal as you can, focusing on eating lean meats, proteins, fruits and vegetables, as appropriate within your diet. If you have any wounds on your skin, make sure you get enough protein, since it is the building-block for new skin.

- *Go at a safe pace.* Don't try to go faster than your body will allow you. During acute rehabilitation, your team will ask you to do exercise that requires your body to perform at its highest level of functioning, but not more. You may feel like you have it in you to walk across your room independently

symptoms of burnout, caregiver burden, stress, anxiety, and depression. Symptoms you should watch for include:

Depression

- Depressed (sad) mood most of the day, almost every day
- Diminished interest or pleasure in activities most of the day, almost every day
- Significant unintentional weight loss or weight gain
- Having others tell you that you're moving, thinking, or speaking more slowly than normal
- Loss of energy nearly every day
- Feeling worthless or bad about yourself (which can appear in thoughts like, "I'm letting myself/my family down")
- Difficulty concentrating
- Thoughts of death, suicide, or wishing you were dead

Anxiety

- Excessive worry or fear
- Difficulties controlling your worries
- Feeling restless, "keyed up" or "on edge"
- Irritability
- Muscle tension
- Difficulty sleeping

Caregiver Burden

- Feeling burdened by taking care of your loved one
- Feeling like your loved one asks for more help than they need

- Feeling stressed between caring for your loved one and meeting your other responsibilities (work, school, parenting)
- Feeling your loved one is dependent on you
- Feeling like you've lost control of your life

Burnout

- Physical or emotional exhaustion
- Feeling cynical or detached
- Feeling like you're ineffective or can't do anything right

If you are experiencing any of these symptoms, it is critical that you seek support. In fact, it is critical that you seek support even if you don't have these symptoms. Support is necessary to prevent mental health concerns. Try support in the form of:

- Calling a friend or family member to "vent"
- Reach out to your psychiatrist, psychologist, or therapist
- Make an appointment with a mental health professional
- Look on Facebook, Reddit, or other online communities for pages/forums related to COVID-19 survival and support (like the Reddit page "COVID19_Support" or the Facebook groups "Covid-19 Support Group", "Survivor Corps" and "COVID-19 Long-Haulers Discussion Group").
- For older adults, the AARP has created a website where you can search for support groups and other forms of help at www.aarpcommunityconnections.org
- Seek counseling from a pastor or minister, if faith is important to you

"I'm so thankful for the [Facebook] group we are in."
- Victoria

It's also important that you continue to do self-care. Don't forget to:

- Avoid excessive alcohol or use of drugs
- Continue to get good sleep
- Prioritize good nutrition
- Continue to do your hobbies or other valued activities—don't let caregiving become the only thing you do
- Socialize (safely) with people other than your loved one

Getting ready to go home

Once you and your team decide that you will be going home, prepare to make the transition from the hospital to home. This is an exciting but daunting time. Here's how you can ensure a safe and manageable transition:

- ***Ask for the anticipated discharge date.*** If you have a whiteboard in your room, ask a nurse to write the date in big letters. This date isn't usually set in stone and might move slightly, depending on progress. But it will give you a general sense of what to expect so you can stay motivated.
- ***Start learning what kind of care you'll need.*** Even if you can't do all your care yourself, learn the steps yourself, if possible, so you can direct family and friends who are helping you. Learn what you can do by yourself and start practicing it.
- ***Discuss any unique features of your home.*** Let your team

know about things like narrow hallways or stairs, so they can help you figure out how to get around at home easily.

- *Ask for printouts.* Gather data sheets about your diet, at-home exercises, and medications. Keep them in a folder or give them to family to keep in a folder for you.
- *Ask about equipment.* Ask your therapists if they recommend any equipment that might help you do what you need to do around the house as you continue to heal. Equipment might include a wheelchair, walker, cane, special grab bars for the bathroom, benches for your shower or tub, etc.
- *Find out which providers you should see after you leave the hospital.* Also ask your case manager to help you set up appointments in advance.
- *Ask if you will need follow-up care with a neuropsychologist.* If you experienced changes in your thinking—and if you plan to return to work, school, or any other activity that requires a lot of thinking and planning—you may need to see a neuropsychologist. The neuropsychologist will evaluate all the areas of your thinking (memory, attention, processing speed, etc.) and give you a sense of how well you're recovering, and what strengths and weaknesses you have. They will also give you a list of recommendations about recovering brain function and compensating for any new weaknesses. You can then take this list to your employer or school so they can provide the necessary accommodations under the ADA law (see next bullet point).
- *Ask your team for any letters you need for your job or school.* Search the internet for "disability rights" and the name of your state for local organizations that can help you understand your rights under the Americans with Disabilities Act, or the ADA. You may have protections for your job

is now negative for COVID-19, or if they are still testing positive. Generally, patients are not discharged until they are negative for COVID-19, but sometimes policies change in times of crisis.

- *Clear pathways.* If your loved one is having any difficulty walking, or is using a wheelchair, cane or walker, remove any area rugs that could be a tripping hazard. You can also tape down edges of rugs with duct tape.
- *Throw a party.* On the day of discharge, plan a small, low-key celebration. Hang balloons, signs, or have a cake (if it's OK on your loved one's diet).

Rehabilitation can be a long journey. The good news is that you are finally leaving the hospital! Yes, you may need to modify your living space. You may need help getting around. You may even need help with everyday tasks. But make sure you take time to celebrate how far you have come and give yourself credit for all that you have accomplished up to this point. And know that when you and loved ones have taken the preparations outlined in this chapter, your transition will be less stressful, more supportive, and will get you closer to a full recovery more quickly.

8

Restarting your Life

Maybe you were hospitalized and went through acute rehabilitation. Maybe you were hospitalized but discharged straight home. Or, maybe you were never hospitalized at all, but are experiencing long-term symptoms of COVID-19. No matter what your story is, well after you have survived the initial infection and possibly even after you have completed rehabilitation therapies, you may still have symptoms that affect your daily function and quality of life. This is a time to both ask for help when you need it (or just want it!), and also a time to continue to focus on your recovery so you can get back to activities you love. Just know that if you have made it this far, you have already proven that you can do anything. And, at the end of this chapter, you will have a clear idea of how to start the process of returning to a life you love, or maybe even building a new life you love even more.

"My scariest moments are when I wake up and can't breathe. Thankfully I have my tiny nebulizer close and can use it to help open my airway. I am thankful to my

*in-laws who went shopping and to the pharmacy for us
when we needed something."*
- Bethann

Starting low and slow at home

Whether you've recently returned from the hospital, or if you were at home all along, taking recovery "low and slow" is critical. Your body has just fought a major battle, and it is common to feel fatigued, short of breath with exertion, "foggy" headed, and maybe even depressed and/or anxious.

If you were never in the hospital, or if you discharged straight home without acute rehabilitation, you may still want to talk to your physician about the option of attending rehabilitation therapies as an outpatient. In order for insurance to cover these therapies, you would need to get a referral from your physician indicating that it is medically necessary and have the necessary therapy coverage on your health plan.

If you do qualify for outpatient rehabilitation, it's well worth considering it as an option. Not only will you get access to dedicated physical and occupational therapists, but if needed you can see a speech-language pathologist as well. These trained professionals can put you through scientifically backed exercises to improve your functioning and teach strategies for what you want to do irrespective of current functioning. They can also send you home with home exercise programs you can do between sessions to help speed your recovery along even more. To learn more about the rehabilitation process, flip back to Chapter 7.

*"It took another month of many small walks for 5-10
minutes to regain my strength in my legs."*
- Jeness

If physical rehabilitation isn't available to you, wasn't necessary,
or if you don't think that it is a good fit, you can still get in
touch with a health or rehabilitation psychologist to help talk
you through adjustment to your new normal. If you have
mental health care covered by insurance, this is a perfect time
to make use of those benefits. You can find a psychologist at
www.locator.apa.org.

Whatever you do, it is important that you listen to your body.
It can be hard to walk the fine line between challenging your
body so that you can get stronger and ignoring critical signals
that it's time to stop. Rehabilitation therapists can help you
find that balance by monitoring your oxygen saturation so you
can get a sense of how far you can "push." But if you're on your
own at home, it can be harder to balance challenging yourself
with good self-care.

If you're recovering at home, signs that it's time to give yourself
a break include:

- Sharp, sudden pain
- Gasping for air/air hunger
- Feeling emotionally overwhelmed, crying, or feeling ex-
  hausted
- Collapsing or experiencing a failure during an exercise
  (falling, dropping equipment, etc.)

Signs that you might be able to "push" include:

- Returning to work
- Re-joining a sports team
- Driving
- Running errands
- Cooking/cleaning
- Volunteering
- Shopping
- Dancing
- Attending social events or church

Now, rank each of the activities you've listed on a low-medium-high scale in terms of how much they require your physical, mental, and emotional capacity. You can use the "Daily Routine Planner" worksheet at www.abigailhardinphd.com to assist with this.

Take getting back to work for example. If you work at a desk job, the physical demands of your work may be pretty minimal, but the mental demands of the job might be quite high. The emotional demands of the job, like collaborating with colleagues, might be somewhere in the middle. In order to successfully transition back to work, you will need to have some minimal to moderate physical capabilities, but just because you can physically sit in your chair to work does not mean you're ready mentally or emotionally.

Another example might be driving your car. Although driving once you're in the car involves some physical capacities (pressing the pedals and sitting upright), it requires a tremendous amount of mental capacity to carefully pay attention, navigate around town, and stay alert. If you're feeling "foggy" mentally, driving is incredibly unsafe.

Once you know what activities you want to get back into

and what capabilities you will need for each of them, figure out which symptom category or categories you need to work on most: weakness, thinking changes, and emotional changes. Then, you can structure your recovery exercises such that they support you returning to these valued activities. It is easy to focus too much on one or another of these categories, but don't forget, you are a whole person, with a brain, emotions and physical capacities. Many patients have a tendency to focus just on physical skills but forget that even if they are physically able to do something, that doesn't mean it will be safe if their brains and emotions can't keep up.

After you've completed the exercise above, you'll be ready to start organizing activities that can help you recover in the areas you think are most important. Below, you will find a list of recovery exercise options for each of the three symptom categories: physical weakness, thinking changes, and emotional changes.

Weakness

- *Go to therapy sessions.* Participate in physical therapy and occupational therapy.
- *Extend your therapies at home.* Do the exercises you are given in your home exercise programs.
- *Get good nutrition.* Lean proteins and plenty of fruits/veggies will help you rebuild muscle faster than junk foods.
- *Consider using daily tasks for exercise.* Try standing on one leg while you brush your teeth (if your PT approves) or take an extra lap around your living room as you're turning off the lights for the night.

- *Ask for a driving evaluation.* If you are planning to return to driving, and you had significant weakness, ask your occupational therapist for a driving evaluation. They will ensure you can physically manage a car and will also help assess whether your reaction speed is fast enough to drive safely.

- *Start daily exercises.* Start exercising a little bit every day, even if it only involves walking around your house or tidying up for five minutes. Build up slowly, starting with five minutes, and adding on a few minutes each day. Once you're ready, try going outside (with a mask) and making a lap around the block, if it's safe.

- *Follow up with physicians.* Go to any follow-up appointments that were recommend to you and address physical concerns with your team. Be sure to mention barriers that are preventing you from doing what you want to do. Barriers can include pain, breathlessness, poor sleep, numbness, weakness in a specific part of your body, etc. Ask if there are any medications, procedures or referrals that they recommend.

- *Find workarounds.* Is there an activity you would like to do, but can't do just yet? While you continue strengthening, see if there's a workaround. For instance, if you love to cook elaborate meals but can't tolerate standing in the kitchen the entire time, try bringing in a stool and taking breaks to sit as you go. Or, if you love running along the lake, but aren't able to go jogging again yet, try moving from bench to bench, taking breaks as you need to.

Thinking Changes

- **Go to therapy sessions.** Participate in speech therapy sessions/cognitive rehabilitation, if these are available to you.
- **Do what you can.** Even if there are activities you can't do entirely on your own, do the parts you can do (like helping navigate while you're a passenger in the car, or organizing the mail even if you're not back to paying the bills yourself just yet).
- **Keep your brain active.** Challenge yourself by trying to read, do puzzles, or even just keep up with current events.
- **Keep a daily agenda.** Take notes on what you do each day so you can look back on it later. Your daily agenda can also help you ensure you don't miss appointments.
- **Use technology.** Use phone alarms, watch alarms, or other devices to help you keep track of times to take your medications, etc.
- **Request a neuropsychology evaluation.** If you're planning to go back to work, school, or driving and you had any significant thinking changes, make an appointment to see a neuropsychologist. Give yourself a few weeks, or even a few months, before you set this appointment to give yourself some time to heal. The neuropsychologist will help you identify the current strengths and weaknesses in your thinking and give you a list of recommendations for how best to return to work or school. If you need ADA accommodations, you can use your neuropsychology report to get them.

9

Thriving after COVID-19

This book has mostly been about a journey related to surviving and overcoming the symptoms of COVID-19. In fact, if that's all that's important to you, you can stop reading here and move on. But this book goes further, and there is a good reason.

Life doesn't just boil down to the daily activities we like to do, or our jobs, or our physical capabilities. Life is also about constructing meaning and living in a way that is consistent with our values even in the face of serious challenges. Surviving COVID-19 is a lot like surviving a car crash, the death of a family member, or other forms of traumatic life events that suddenly shatter your perspective of your life and yourself and force you to build up a new mindset from scratch. Thriving after any kind of serious life event involves not just returning to the day-to-day activities that make up your life (your job, paying bills, your hobbies, etc.), but finding a mindset that allows you to build a new life once your old one has been shattered.

In this last chapter, you will learn how to make sense of what you have been through and how to construct a life you love even more than the one you had before your battle with COVID-19.

Living with ongoing symptoms

After you have survived COVID-19, and even after you have completed your rehabilitation program, it is possible you might have long-term symptoms. If you had complications during your hospitalization like a stroke, heart attack, or loss of oxygen to the brain, some of these changes can be permanent. Even if it has been a long time since you survived COVID-19, it's never a problem to have hope that you will continue to recover, gain function, or at the very least, learn strategies that will continue to make you feel more independent.

> *"As for the long haul? I think I'm finally better now. I'm not at 100% as strenuous activity tires me pretty quickly, but the smell is gone and I no longer get foggy headed. My energy comes back a little more every day."*
> - Matt

Whether you are living with permanent symptoms, or simply continuing to work on improving your function and independence, don't put your life on hold simply because you're not "back to where you were" before you got sick.

Do something you enjoy

Don't focus exclusively on your symptoms. Remember, you are a survivor. You have been focusing on your COVID-19 infection for a very long time. It's sort of like staring at your computer screen for too long in the dark and realizing you can't and I wish you the best of health and happiness in the "chapters" to come.

If you are a survivor, I offer you my congratulations, and encourage you to reach out to other COVID-19 survivors to offer your support and words of wisdom. The COVID-19 pandemic is truly unprecedented in the stresses, losses, and fear it has caused. The only way I know how to combat COVID-19's effects is by writing this book and hopefully helping you survive and thrive. Find your way to fight the pandemic now as a survivor, by providing support, advice and comfort to those around you.

I ask that if this book has been helpful to you, you do something for me in return. Please pass along your support and compassion to others. You can recommend this book to them if you would like. But at the very least, please reach out with kindness, compassion and support to your friends, family and neighbors. We are all in this together.

Good luck out there and be well.

Join other survivors and healthcare professionals who have signed up to receive my free newsletter at www.abigailhardinphd.com. By signing up, you'll get free access to printable versions of all the resources and worksheets mentioned in this book, as well as updates and exclusive content on COVID-19 and rehabilitation.

References

1. Pneumonia of unknown cause - China. World Health Organization. https://www.who.int/csr/don/05-january-2020-pneumonia-of-unkown-cause-china/en/. Published January 5, 2020. Accessed August 8, 2020.
2. Singhal T. A Review of Coronavirus Disease-2019 (COVID-19). *Indian J Pediatr*. 2020;87(April):281-286.
3. Rothe C, Schunk M, Sothmann P, et al. Transmission of 2019-NCOV infection from an asymptomatic contact in Germany. *N Engl J Med*. 2020;382(10):970-971. doi:10.1056/NEJMc2001468
4. Cheng ZJ, Shan J. 2019 Novel coronavirus: where we are and what we know. *Infection*. 2020;48(2):155-163. doi:10.1007/s15010-020-01401-y
5. Mortality Analaysis. Johns Hopkins Coronavirus Resource Center. https://coronavirus.jhu.edu/data/mortality. Updated September 16, 2020. Accessed September 16, 2020.
6. Huang C, Wang Y, Li X, et al. Clinical features of patients infected with 2019 novel coronavirus in Wuhan, China. *Lancet*. 2020;395(10223):497-506. doi:10.1016/S0140-6736(20)30183-5
7. Moein ST, Hashemian SMR, Mansourafshar B, Khorram-Tousi A, Tabarsi P, Doty RL. Smell dysfunction: a

biomarker for COVID-19. *Int Forum Allergy Rhinol.* 2020;10(8):944-950. doi:10.1002/alr.22587

8. Halpin SJ, McIvor C, Whyatt G, et al. Post-discharge symptoms and rehabilitation needs in survivors of COVID-19 infection: a cross-sectional evaluation. *J Med Virol.* 2020;n/a(n/a):0-2. doi:10.1002/jmv.26368

9. Carfi A, Bernabei R, Landi F.Persistent Symptoms in Patients After Acute COVID-19. *JAMA.* 2020;324(6):603-605. doi:10.1001/jama.2020.12603

10. Mazza MG, De Lorenzo R, Conte C, et al. Anxiety and depression in COVID-19 survivors: Role of inflammatory and clinical predictors. *Brain Behav Immun.* 2020;(July):1-7. doi:10.1016/j.bbi.2020.07.037

11. Zhou F, Yu T, Du R, et al. Clinical course and risk factors for mortality of adult inpatients with COVID-19 in Wuhan, China: a retrospective cohort study. *Lancet.* 2020;395(10229):1054-1062. doi:10.1016/S0140-6736(20)30566-3

12. Gao F, Zheng KI, Wang XB, et al. Obesity Is a Risk Factor for Greater COVID-19 Severity. *Diabetes Care.* 2020;43(7):E72-E74. doi:10.2337/dc20-0682

13. Wu Z, McGoogan JM. Characteristics of and Important Lessons from the Coronavirus Disease 2019 (COVID-19) Outbreak in China: Summary of a Report of 72314 Cases from the Chinese Center for Disease Control and Prevention. *JAMA - J Am Med Assoc.* 2020;323(13):1239-1242. doi:10.1001/jama.2020.2648

14. Facts About Hypertension. cdc.gov. https://www.cdc.gov-/bloodpressure/facts.htm. Published 2020. Accessed November 8, 2020.

15. Hales CM, Carroll MD, Fryar CD, Ogden CL. Prevalence

of Obesity and Severe Obesity Among Adults: United States, 2017-2018. *NCHS Data Brief.* 2020;(360):1-8.

16. How to Protect Yourself & Others. cdc.gov. www.cdc.gov /coronavirus/2019-ncov/prevent-getting-sick /prevention.html. Published 2020. Accessed December 8, 2020.

17. Shields GS, Sazma MA, Yonelinas AP. The effects of acute stress on core executive functions: A meta-analysis and comparison with cortisol. *Neurosci Biobehav Rev.* 2016;68:651-668. doi:10.1016/j.neubiorev.2016.06.038

18. People with Certain Medical Conditions. cdc.gov. https://www.cdc.gov/coronavirus/2019-ncov/need-extra-precautions/people-with-medical-conditions.html. Updated September 11, 2020. Accessed September 16, 2020.

19. Cohen S, Tyrrell DA, Russell MA, Jarvis MJ, Smith AP. Smoking, alcohol consumption, and susceptibility to the common cold. *Am J Public Health.* 1993;83(9):1277-1283. doi:10.2105/AJPH.83.9.1277

20. Grundy EJ, Suddek T, Filippidis FT, Majeed A, Coronini-Cronberg S. Smoking, SARS-CoV-2 and COVID-19: A review of reviews considering implications for public health policy and practice. *Tob Induc Dis.* 2020;18:58. doi:10.18332/tid/124788

21. Myles IA. Fast food fever: reviewing the impacts of the Western diet on immunity. *Nutr J.* 2014;13(1):61. doi:10.1186/1475-2891-13-61

22. Barrea L, Muscogiuri G, Frias-Toral E, et al. Nutrition and immune system: from the Mediterranean diet to dietary supplementary through the microbiota. *Crit Rev Food Sci Nutr.* Published online July 21, 2020:1-25. doi:10.1080/10408398.2020.1792826

23. Calatayud FM, Calatayud B, Gallego JG, González-Martín C, Alguacil LF. Effects of Mediterranean diet in patients with recurring colds and frequent complications. *Allergol Immunopathol (Madr).* 2017;45(5):417-424. doi:https://-doi.org/10.1016/j.aller.2016.08.006

24. Pasala S, Barr T, Messaoudi I. Impact of Alcohol Abuse on the Adaptive Immune System. *Alcohol Res.* 2015;37(2):185-197.

25. Testino G. Are Patients With Alcohol Use Disorders at Increased Risk for Covid-19 Infection? *Alcohol Alcohol.* 2020;55(4):344-346. doi:10.1093/alcalc/agaa037

26. Dietary Guidelines for Alcohol. cdc.gov. www.cdc.gov /alcohol/fact-sheets/moderate-drinking.htm. Published December 30, 2019. Accessed September 14, 2020

27. Irwin MR. Why Sleep Is Important for Health: A Psychoneuroimmunology Perspective. *Annu Rev Psychol.* 2015;66(1):143-172. doi:10.1146/annurev-psych-010213-115205

28. Besedovsky L, Lange T, Born J. Sleep and immune function. *Pflügers Arch - Eur J Physiol.* 2012;463(1):121-137. doi:10.1007/s00424-011-1044-0

29. Roehrs T, Yoon J, Roth T. Nocturnal and next-day effects of ethanol and basal level of sleepiness. *Hum Psychopharmacol Clin Exp.* 1991;6(4):307-311.

30. Shields GS, Spahr CM, Slavich GM. Psychosocial Interventions and Immune System Function: A Systematic Review and Meta-analysis of Randomized Clinical Trials. *JAMA Psychiatry.* Published online June 3, 2020. doi:10.1001/jamapsychiatry.2020.0431

31. Uchino BN, Trettevik R, Kent de Grey RG, Cronan S, Hogan J, Baucom BRW. Social support, social integration,

and inflammatory cytokines: A meta-analysis. *Heal Psychol.* 2018;37(5):462-471. doi:10.1037/hea0000594

32. Pedersen BK, Hoffman-Goetz L. Exercise and the Immune System: Regulation, Integration,and Adaptation. *Physiol Rev.* 2000;80(3):1055-1081. doi:10.1152/physrev.2000.80.3.1055

33. How Much Physical Activity Do Adults Need? cdc.gov. https://www.cdc.gov/physicalactivity/basics/adults/index.htm. Updated May 14, 2020. Accessed September 14, 2020.

34. Campos P. *The Obesity Myth: Why America's Obsession with Weight Is Hazardous to Your Health.* Gotham Books; 2004. doi:10.1093/ije/dyi052

35. Gaesser G. *Big Fat Lies.* Gurze Books; 2002.

36. Bacon L, Aphramor L. Weight Science: Evaluating the Evidence for a Paradigm Shift. *Nutr J.* 2011;10(1):9. doi:10.1186/1475-2891-10-9

37. Bailey P, Thomsen GE, Spuhler VJ, et al. Early activity is feasible and safe in respiratory failure patients. *Crit Care Med.* 2007;35(1). https://journals.lww.com/ccmjournal/Fulltext/2007/01000/Early_activity_is_feasible_and_safe_in_respiratory.22.aspx

38. Treating COVID-19 at home: Care tips for you and others. mayoclinic.org. https://www.mayoclinic.org/diseases-conditions/coronavirus/in-depth/treating-covid-19-at-home/art-20483273. Updated September 15, 2020. Accessed September 14, 2020.

39. Dantzer R, O'Connor JC, Freund GG, Johnson RW, Kelley KW. From inflammation to sickness and depression: when the immune system subjugates the brain. *Nat Rev Neurosci.* 2008;9(1):46-56. doi:10.1038/nrn2297

40. Toda H, Williams JA, Gulledge M, Sehgal A. A sleep-inducing gene, nemuri, links sleep and immune function in Drosophila.*Science.* 2019;363(6426):509-515.

41. van den Brink GR, van den Boogaardt DEM, van Deventer SJH, Peppelenbosch MP. Feed a cold, starve a fever? *Clin Diagn Lab Immunol.* 2002;9(1):182-183. doi:10.1128/cdli.9.1.182-183.2002

42. Saketkhoo K, Januszkiewicz A, Sackner MA. Effects of Drinking Hot Water, Cold Water, and Chicken Soup on Nasal Mucus Velocity and Nasal Airflow Resistance. *Chest.* 1978;74(4):408-410. doi:10.1016/S0012-3692(15)37387-6

43. D'Souza NB, Bagby GJ, Nelson S, Lang CH, Spitzer JJ. Acute Alcohol Infusion Suppresses Endotoxin-induced Serum Tumor Necrosis Factor. *Alcohol Clin Exp Res.* 1989;13(2):295-298.

44. Guppy MPB, Mickan SM, Del Mar CB, Thorning S, Rack A. Advising patients to increase fluid intake for treating acute respiratory infections. *Cochrane Database Syst Rev.* 2011;(2). doi:10.1002/14651858.CD004419.pub3

45. World Health Organization. *Home care for patients with suspected or confirmed COVID-19 and and management of their contacts.* World Health Organization; 2020.

46. Symptoms. cdc.gov. https://www.cdc.gov/coronavirus/2019-ncov/symptoms-testing/symptoms.html. Published 2020. Accessed November 8, 2020.

47. Murthy S, Gomersall CD, Fowler RA. Care for Critically Ill Patients with COVID-19. *JAMA - J Am Med Assoc.* 2020;323(15):1499-1500. doi:10.1001/jama.2020.3633

48. Pelosi P, Croci M, Calappi E, et al. Prone positioning improves pulmonary function in obese patients during

general anesthesia. *Anesth Analg.* 1996;83(3):578-583. doi:10.1097/00000539-199609000-00025

49. White A, Fan E, Ventetuolo CE, Kulkarni H, Carmona MS, Sockrider M. What is ECMO? *Am J Respir Crit Care Med.* 2016;193(6):P9-P10. doi:10.1164/rccm.1936P9

50. Pun BT, Ely EW. The Importance of Diagnosing and Managing ICU Delirium. *Chest.* 2007;132(2):624-636. doi:https://doi.org/10.1378/chest.06-1795

51. McGowan SK, Behar E. A Preliminary Investigation of Stimulus Control Training for Worry: Effects on Anxiety and Insomnia. *Behav Modif.* 2012;37(1):90-112. doi:10.1177/0145445512455661

52. Preparing Children for Visiting the Hospital. Johns Hopkins Childrens Center. https://www.hopkins-medicine.org/johns-hopkins-childrens-center/what-we-treat/specialties/palliative-care/grief-bereavement/sibling-young-children-support/preparing-children-visiting-hospital.html. Accessed August 12, 2020.

53. Mangalmurti N, Hunter CA. Cytokine Storms: Understanding COVID-19. *Immunity.* 2020;53(1):19-25. doi:10.1016/j.immuni.2020.06.017

54. Inoue S, Hatakeyama J, Kondo Y, et al. Post-intensive care syndrome: its pathophysiology, prevention, and future directions. *Acute Med Surg.* Published online 2019:233-246. doi:10.1002/ams2.415

55. Marra A, Pandharipande P, Girard T, et al. Co-occurrence of Post-Intensive Care Syndrome Problems Among 406 Survivors of Critical Illness. *Crit Care Med.* 2018;46(9):1393-1401.

56. Hodgson C, Bellomo R, Berney S, et al. Early mobilization and recovery in mechanically ventilated patients in the

ICU: A bi-national, multi-centre, prospective cohort study. *Crit Care.* 2015;19(1):1-10. doi:10.1186/s13054-015-0765-4

57. Tingey JL, Bentley JA, Hosey MM. COVID-19: Understanding and Mitigating Trauma in ICU Survivors. *Psychol Trauma Theory, Res Pract Policy.* 2020;12:100-104. doi:10.1037/tra0000884

58. Puthucheary ZA, Rawal J, McPhail M, et al. Acute Skeletal Muscle Wasting in Critical Illness. *JAMA.* 2013;310(15):1591-1600. doi:10.1001/jama.2013.278481

59. Macht M, King CJ, Wimbish T, et al. Post-extubation dysphagia is associated with longer hospitalization in survivors of critical illness with neurologic impairment. *Dysphagia.* 2014;29(1):118-119. doi:10.1007/s00455-013-9492-7

60. Kotfis K, Williams Roberson S, Wilson JE, Dabrowski W, Pun BT, Ely EW. COVID-19: ICU delirium management during SARS-CoV-2 pandemic. *Crit Care.* 2020;24(1):1-9. doi:10.1186/s13054-020-02882-x

61. Brummel NE, Jackson JC, Pandharipande PP, et al. Delirium in the ICU and subsequent long-term disability among survivors of mechanical ventilation. *Crit Care Med.* 2014;42(2):369-377.

62. Hopkins RO, Weaver LK, Collingridge D, Parkinson RB, Chan KJ, Orme JF. Two-year cognitive, emotional, and quality-of-life outcomes in acute respiratory distress syndrome. *Am J Respir Crit Care Med.* 2005;171(4):340-347. doi:10.1164/rccm.200406-763OC

63. Jackson JC, Pandharipande PP, Girard TD, et al. Depression, post-traumatic stress disorder, and functional disability in survivors of critical illness in the BRAIN-

ICU study: a longitudinal cohort study. *Lancet Respir Med.* 2014;2(5):369-379.

64. Jones C, Bäckman C, Capuzzo M, et al. Intensive care diaries reduce new onset post traumatic stress disorder following critical illness: A randomised, controlled trial. *Crit Care.* 2010;14(5). doi:10.1186/cc9260

65. Puntmann VO, Carerj ML, Wieters I, et al. Outcomes of Cardiovascular Magnetic Resonance Imaging in Patients Recently Recovered From Coronavirus Disease 2019 (COVID-19). *JAMA Cardiol.* Published online July 27, 2020. doi:10.1001/jamacardio.2020.3557

66. Vincent JL, Taccone FS. Understanding pathways to death in patients with COVID-19. *Lancet Respir Med.* 2020;8(5):430-432. doi:10.1016/S2213-2600(20)30165-X

67. Zaim S, Chong JH, Sankaranarayanan V, Harky A. COVID-19 and Multiorgan Response. *Curr Probl Cardiol.* 2020;45(8):100618. doi:10.1016/j.cpcardiol.2020.100618

68. Simpson R, Robinson L. Rehabilitation After Critical Illness in People With COVID-19 Infection. *Am J Phys Med Rehabil.* 2020;99(6):470-474.

69. Heinemann AW, Wilson CS, Huston T, et al. Relationship of psychology inpatient rehabilitation services and patient characteristics to outcomes following spinal cord injury: The SCIRehab Project. *J Spinal Cord Med.* 2012;35(6):578-592.

70. Kortte KB, Stevenson JE, Hosey MM, Castillo R, Wegener ST. Hope predicts positive functional role outcomes in acute rehabilitation populations. *Rehabil Psychol.* 2012;57(3):248-255. doi:10.1037/a0029004

71. Kennedy P, Lude P, Elfstrm ML, Smithson EF. Psychological contributions to functional independence:

A longitudinal investigation of spinal cord injury rehabilitation. *Arch Phys Med Rehabil.* 2011;92(4):597-602. doi:10.1016/j.apmr.2010.11.016

72. Tedeschi RG, Park CL, Calhoun LG. *Posttraumatic Growth: Positive Changes in the Aftermath of Crisis.* (Weiner IB, ed.). Lawrence Erlbaum Associates, Inc.; 1998.

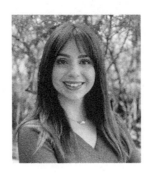

About the Author

Abigail S. Hardin is a licensed clinical psychologist in the specialty practice area of rehabilitation psychology. She specializes in working with people who have sustained catastrophic illnesses and injuries, with a particular emphasis on those who have survived ICU admissions. She has been providing direct care to COVID-19 patients since the beginning of the pandemic, including follow-up care months after their hospital discharge. Dr. Hardin also provides psychological care to staff within the COVID-19 ICU and acute floors as a part of her University's Wellness Response Team.

Dr. Hardin has worked in some of the best hospitals and rehabilitation centers in the U.S., including TIRR Memorial Hermann (ranked the third best rehabilitation hospital in the States), the University of Washington, and Rush University Medical Center in Chicago, IL.

Dr. Hardin earned a Ph.D. in clinical health psychology and an M.A. in psychology from the University of North Carolina Charlotte, plus a B.A. in public relations and psychology from the University of Southern California.

You can connect with me on:
- http://www.abigailhardinphd.com
- https://twitter.com/AHardinPhD
- https://www.facebook.com/abigailhardinphd

Made in the USA
Monee, IL
20 January 2021